ADDISON'S DISEASE
PATIENT ADVOCATE

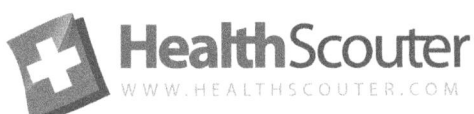

HealthScouter.com - Equity Press
5055 Canyon Crest Drive
Riverside, California 92507

www.healthscouter.com

Purchasing this book entitles you to free updates
at www.healthscouter.com/Addison'sDisease

Edited By: Katrina Robinson

Includes Addison's Disease from Wikipedia http://en.wikipedia.org/wiki/Addison'sDisease

HealthScouter Addison's Disease: Addison Disease Symptoms and Addison's Disease Treatment (HealthScouter Addison's Disease)

ISBN 978-1-60332-118-1

Edited components are copyright ©2009 Equity Press and HealthScouter all rights reserved.

Permission is granted to copy, distribute, and/or modify this document under the terms of the GNU Free Documentation License, Version 1.2 or any later version published by the Free Software Foundation; with no Invariant Sections, no Front-Cover Texts, and no Back-Cover Texts. A copy of the license is included in the section entitled "GNU Free Documentation License."

Trademarks: All trademarks are the property of their respective owners. Equity Press is not associated with any product or vendor mentioned in this book.

Important

NEVER DISREGARD PROFESSIONAL MEDICAL ADVICE, OR DELAY SEEKING IT, BECAUSE OF SOMETHING YOU HAVE READ IN THIS BOOK. ALWAYS SEEK PROFESSIONAL MEDICAL ADVICE BEFORE ACTING UPON INFORMATION READ IN THIS BOOK.

HealthScouter and Equity Press do not provide medical advice. The contents of this book are for informational purposes only and are not intended to substitute for professional medical advice, diagnosis or treatment. Always seek advice from a qualified physician or health care professional about any medical concern, and do not disregard professional medical advice because of anything you may read in this book or on a HealthScouter Web site. The views of individuals quoted in this book are not necessarily those of HealthScouter or Equity Press.

While this book is intended to be a medium for the exchange of information and ideas, it is not meant in any way to be a substitute for sound medical advice; neither should it be viewed as a trusted source of such advice. The views expressed in these messages are not those of any qualified medical association, and the publisher is not responsible for the validity of the information communicated herein or for consequences that may arise from acting upon this information. The publisher is not responsible for any content found in the book that may be deemed offensive, inappropriate, inaccurate or medically unsound. The information you find here is only for the purpose of discussion and should not be the basis for any medical decision. The content is not intended to be a substitute for professional medical advice, diagnosis or treatment.

The information presented is not to be considered complete, nor does it contain all medical resource information that may be relevant, and therefore it is not intended to be a substitute for seeking medical treatment and/or appropriate care.

By reading this book and parts of the Web site, you agree under all circumstances to hold harmless, and to refrain from seeking remedy from, the owners of this book. The publisher shall disclaim all liability to you for damages, costs or expenses, including legal and medical fees, related to your reliance on anything derived from this book or Web site or its contents. Furthermore, Equity Press assumes no liability for any and all claims arising out of the said use, regardless of the cause, effects, or fault.

Equity Press and HealthScouter do not endorse any company or product, and listing on the HealthScouter Web site is not linked to corporate sponsorship. We do not make a claim to being comprehensive or up to date. If you would like to recommend information to include in this book, please contact us – we would be very happy to hear from you.

Purchasing this book entitles you to free updates as they are available. Please register your book at www.healthscouter.com

TABLE OF CONTENTS

Introduction and Motivation 6

How to Use This Book 12

Introduction to Addison's Disease 15

Symptoms 19
    Clinical signs 20
    Addisonian crisis 22

Diagnosis 27
    Suggestive features 27
    Testing 29

Causes 33
    Adrenal dysgenesis 33
    Impaired steroidogenesis 33
    Adrenal destruction 34

Treatment 37
    Maintenance treatment 37

Epidemiology 39

Prognosis 41

Canine Hypoadrenocorticism 45

Adrenal Insufficiency 47
    Types 49
    Causes 51
    Symptoms 52
    Diagnosis 54
    Treatment 54

Adrenocorticotropic Hormone Stimulation Test 57
    Versions of the test 59
    Preparation 61
    Administration 62
    Potential side effects 64
    Interpretation of results 64

  Cortisol stimulation. 64
  Adrenocorticotropic hormone plasma test plus cortisol stimulation 66
  Aldosterone stimulation 68
 Other hormones and chemicals that will rise in the adrenocorticotropic hormone
  stimulation test 70

Adrenoleukodystrophy 71
 Symptoms 72
 Diagnosis. 74
 Pathophysiology 74
  X-linked. 74
  Autosomal 75
 Treatment 76
 Prognosis. 77
 Research 78

Adrenomyeloneuropathy 79
 Presentation 80
 Relatives of an Affected Patient 80

Adrenal Fatigue. 83

Autoimmune Adrenalitis. 87

Cortisol 89
 Physiology. 90
 Effects. 92
  Insulin. 92
  Amino acids. 93
  Gastric secretion. 93
  Sodium 94
  Potassium 94
  Water 95
  Copper. 95
  Immune system 96
  Bone metabolism 97
  Memory. 97
  Additional effects 98
 Binding 100

Regulation	100
Factors affecting cortisol levels	102
Factors generally reducing cortisol levels	102
Factors generally increasing cortisol levels	105
Pharmacology	106
Biochemistry	109
Biosynthesis	109
Metabolism	110
References – Addison's Disease	112
References – Adrenal Insufficiency	114
References – Adrenocorticotropic Hormone Stimulation Test	116
References – Adrenoleukydystrophy	118
References – Adrenomyeloneuropathy	122
References – Adrenal Fatigue	124
References – Autoimmune Adrenalitis	126
References – Cortisol	128
GNU Free Documentation License	134
Index	142

INTRODUCTION AND MOTIVATION

Dear Reader,

I like to think of myself as a polite, well-reasoned person. I rarely speak out or complain. When a waitress spills something on me, or if my meal is cold—or if I'm overcharged—I generally try to be as polite as possible. I don't like to make very many waves. I often secretly hope that the manager will hear about my predicament and come out and offer me a free meal, or something similar. I generally hope that my polite and respectful demeanor pays off. And it does happen from time to time. You know, I think many people are brought up to believe that this is just good manners. It's how you're supposed to behave. And if you knew me personally, I think you'd agree that I'm generally pretty reserved. Of course my wife may raise an objection or two (!), but I really believe that it's important to treat others as you would like to be treated. We're talking about the golden rule here—it works well and it applies to almost every life circumstance.

But I have to admit that when it comes to my health, or the health of someone I care about—all bets are off. I want to know what's going on—when, why, where, and how. And I make these feelings known. I tend to get downright assertive. It's just something I feel very strongly about. And I feel that when you are in a hospital, or if you're brushing up against the healthcare system, that you should feel the same way. It's unfamiliar turf, and the professionals who work in this system often take advantage of their positions. They may use some jargon to hide the whole truth— or they may say something without checking to make sure you understand completely. They may present the options that are best for them, perhaps the most profitable or convenient. Now I'm not saying this goes on everywhere. There are many professionals in the business of health who go out of their way to make sure you have the best care. And I'm not suggesting that you should become a bully, or purposefully annoying—absolutely not. But I am suggesting that I think it's OK for you to step outside of your typical comfort zone, and put on your patient advocate hat. Because you, the patient or patient advocate, care the most about your care—not the medical system or healthcare providers.

HealthScouter was created to help patients become better advocates for their own medical care. Because when it comes to your healthcare, the stakes are high. There are none higher. And healthcare is one area where consumers (us, the sick people) are notoriously unaware of their options. And that's why I'm publishing these books. To help you understand your options, and to help you get the best care possible. I want to help you become a better advocate for yourself and for your loved ones.

It's my sincere hope that you can take this book with you to the hospital, to be read in the waiting room or by the bedside—and when you see a relevant patient comment you can use this book to ask questions of your health care providers. My advice: Ask lots of questions! Providers are busy people who generally go about their business with little questioning, delivering care as they see fit—making quick decisions—and again, nobody is going to care as much about your health as you. So now, more than ever, you need tools at your disposal to get the best care possible. One of the tools at your disposal is this HealthScouter book and the material within. You need to be armed with questions, and you need to ask questions all of the time. And so the difficult part is now to understand the right questions to ask.

That brings me to an explanation of how these books are structured. HealthScouter books include a number of what we call patient comments. These patient comments are summaries of what people have experienced. They're first hand accounts of what you may expect. These experiences effectively help you "catch up," and understand what outcomes are possible. They expose you to the treatments are available, and provide insight as to potential outcomes. They help you understand what other people are doing. So if you find yourself stuck feeling like you're receiving substandard medical care—or if you need a push to broach the subject, you can take this book to your provider and say, "Hey, I read here that another patient had this treatment—is that an option for me? If not, Why?" I believe that other peoples' experience is the most valuable way for you to formulate and build a list of good questions for your healthcare providers.

That notion is at the core of the HealthScouter philosophy.

So HealthScouter, by providing patient comments about a particular medical condition, will help expose you to what other people have experienced about a particular medical problem. If you know what other people have experienced, you can better understand what your options are. You'll be better informed and you'll have some questions to ask—it'll be like you've had access to dozens of other people who have gone through the same thing you're going through. And so armed, maybe you'll be able to move through your condition and get back on the road to health, and maybe you'll be able to do this with more grace than I have. And that is my sincere wish.

It's also my wish that perhaps when a doctor or nurse sees this little blue book, that they'll think twice about the care they're about to provide—knowing that the owner is a little bit better prepared, a little bit better armed—and yes, maybe even downright assertive.

I hope this book helps.

Yours truly,

Jim Stewart

San Diego, California

ADDISON'S DISEASE

HOW TO USE THIS BOOK

The purpose of HealthScouter is to help you understand your medical condition as quickly and easily as possible. We believe this can best be accomplished by reading about other people and their experiences negotiating their health and care. We try to leave out complicated medical jargon. And we've spent a considerable amount of time structuring this book so that it's easy to use. It's important to know that this is not the sort of book you read from beginning to end. Of course you may do so, but this book is more meaningful if you flip through quickly and scan for applicable material. Again, it's all about the patient commentary: The darkly shaded comments indicate one patient initiating a new discussion, and the light or clear comments are other comments associated with that same condition. So you should begin by looking for information from other patients who are experiencing the same aspect of the same medical condition that you studying. You can do this quickly by scanning through the book, focusing on the dark shaded comment boxes. By scanning the patient comments you'll find information about various aspects of a condition, all grouped together, in an easy-to-read format. In this way you can immediately begin reading about other patients and their experiences with your particular medical condition – and you can benefit immediately from their experiences.

HEALTHSCOUTER

INTRODUCTION TO ADDISON'S DISEASE

Addison's disease (also known as chronic adrenal insufficiency, hypocortisolism or hypocorticism) is a rare endocrine disorder in which the adrenal gland does not produce enough steroid hormones (glucocorticoids and often mineralocorticoids).[1] It may develop in children, adults or some species of animals, and may occur as the result of many underlying causes.

The condition is named after Dr Thomas Addison, the British physician who first described the condition in his 1849 publication On the Constitutional and Local Effects of Disease of the Suprarenal Capsules.[2] The adjective "Addisonian" is used for features of the condition, as well as patients with Addison's disease.[3]

The condition is generally diagnosed with blood tests, medical imaging and additional investigations.[3] Treatment involves replacement of the hormones (oral hydrocortisone and fludrocortisone). If the disease is caused by an underlying problem, it may be possible to address that. Regular follow-up and monitoring for other health problems is necessary.[3]

While Addison's six patients in 1855 all had adrenal tuberculosis,[4] the term "Addison's disease" does not imply an underlying disease

HEALTHSCOUTER

In June, the doctors diagnosed me with Addison's disease. Now the doctors have told me that they believe I may be suffering with Lyme's disease as well. My condition has gotten much worse since they put me on these steroids for Addison's. Now it has effected my nervous system and the doctors are baffled. They are doing a Lyme's.

Does anyone if it's true that steroids can make Lyme's disease twice as bad? This scares me, as I cannot come off the steroids because of the Addison's disease. Does anyone know how hard it is to get rid of Lyme's disease once it has started to hit the nervous system? Is it curable?

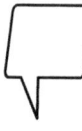
A person can get better if they have Lyme. Not cured but better. I have heard once you have gotten the bacteria in you, you will always have it. The trick is, is to raise the immune system.

I was told I had Addison at one point along my journey. I was told I had many conditions... but I had Lyme. I didn't do treatment for Addison's. I did have a doctor put me on steroids to ease the inflammation and it was the worst thing any doctor could do to a patient. They are NOT good for a person's system.

If the doctors suspect Lyme, they need to treat you for Lyme. They need to put you on antibiotics until your symptoms disappear.

HEALTHSCOUTER

SYMPTOMS

The symptoms of Addison's disease develop insidiously, and it may take some time to be recognized. The most common symptoms are fatigue, dizziness, muscle weakness, weight loss, difficulty in standing up, vomiting, anxiety, diarrhea, headache, sweating, changes in mood and personality, and joint and muscle pains. Some have marked cravings for salt or salty foods due to the urinary losses of sodium.[3] Adrenal insufficiency is manifested in the skin primarily by hyperpigmentation.[5]

A few months ago I learned I have Addison's. Does anyone have problems with pain in their legs, and is it because of Addison's? I am extremely tired and get pains day and night.

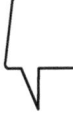

I am also new to Addison's and have pain in my legs, along with lots of fluid, and they feel really weak too. I have been sick with some other pain problems for many years, and have been very inactive for all that time, so I did not have a lot of strength even before I got Addison's. But the leg swelling and the pain came when I started the medicine. I would say, but without knowing much about it, that to me it sounds like you might not get enough medicine if you are so tired.

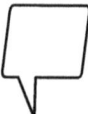 *I have been diagnosed with Addison's. I have been taking hydrocortisone, but it only helps a little. I have to say the pain in my legs and hands started after taking this medicine.*

Clinical signs

Because primary hypocortisolism is manifested as a deficiency in glucocorticoid release from the adrenal cortex, increased adrenocorticotropic hormone will be released by the pituitary in order to trigger release of the absent glucocorticoid; it is because of this overstimulation of adrenocorticotropic hormone that bronzing of the skin occurs. In secondary or tertiary hypocortisolism, there is a deficiency of either corticotropin releasing hormone or adrenocorticotropic hormone release by the hypothalamus or pituitary gland, respectively. The former will manifest as no adrenocorticotropic hormone release while the latter will manifest as physiologic (normal) adrenocorticotropic hormone release; neither will cause an overproduction of adrenocorticotropic hormone.

On examination, the following may be noticed:[3]

- Low blood pressure that falls further when standing (orthostatic hypotension)

ADDISON'S DISEASE

- Most people with primary Addison's have darkening (hyperpigmentation) of the skin, including areas not exposed to the sun; characteristic sites are skin creases (e.g. of the hands), nipples, and the inside of the cheek (buccal mucosa), also old scars may darken. This occurs because melanocyte-stimulating hormone (MSH) shares the same precursor molecule as adrenocorticotropic hormone (ACTH); an increase in adrenocorticotropic hormone production also increases melanocyte-stimulating hormone. In secondary and tertiary forms of Addison's, skin darkening does not occur.

- Signs of conditions that often occur together with Addison's: goiter and vitiligo.

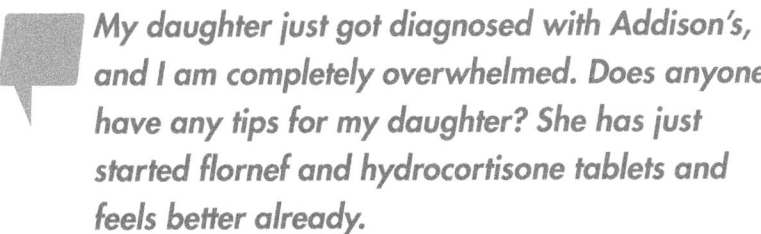

My daughter just got diagnosed with Addison's, and I am completely overwhelmed. Does anyone have any tips for my daughter? She has just started flornef and hydrocortisone tablets and feels better already.

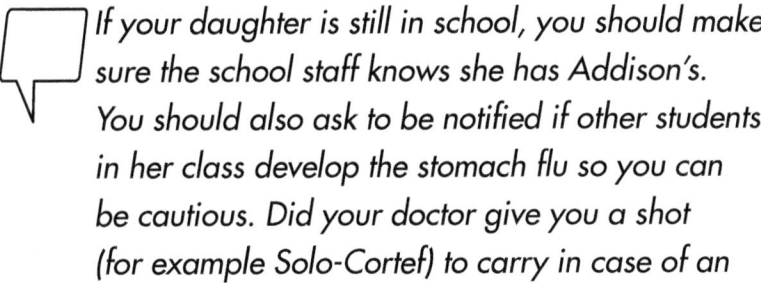

If your daughter is still in school, you should make sure the school staff knows she has Addison's. You should also ask to be notified if other students in her class develop the stomach flu so you can be cautious. Did your doctor give you a shot (for example Solo-Cortef) to carry in case of an

emergency? If your daughter gets the stomach flu, she will need extra medication. For me, I have had several crises because of the stomach flu and have to go to the emergency room shortly after beginning to vomit. She will also need more medication for any type of surgery or if she is in a serious accident. She should wear a medical bracelet.

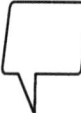*With Addison's, the key is getting the right amount of medications that works for you. Once you have found the right amount you do pretty well. When you get sick, if you cannot keep your medications down, you have to go to the emergency room because you can go into Adrenal shock.*

Addisonian crisis

An "Addisonian crisis" or "adrenal crisis" is a constellation of symptoms that indicate severe adrenal insufficiency. This may be the result of either previously undiagnosed Addison's disease, a disease process suddenly affecting adrenal function (such as adrenal hemorrhage), or an underlying problem (e.g. infection, trauma) in the setting of known Addison's disease. Additionally, this situation may develop in those on long-term oral glucocorticoids who have suddenly ceased taking their medication. In these people, long term use of synthetic glucocorticoids will have caused further atrophy of the adrenal glands by negative feedback. It is also a concern in the setting of myxedema coma; thyroxine given in that setting without glucocorticoids may precipitate a crisis.

Untreated, an Addisonian crisis can be fatal. It is a medical emergency, usually requiring hospitalization. Characteristic symptoms are:[6]

- Sudden penetrating pain in the legs, lower back or abdomen
- Severe vomiting and diarrhea, resulting in dehydration
- Low blood pressure
- Syncope (loss of consciousness)
- Hypoglycemia
- Confusion, psychosis, slurred speech
- Severe lethargy
- Hypocalcaemia
- Convulsions
- Fever

I have had Addison's Disease since 1987 and was put on Cortisone maintenance. I had a very severe Addisonian Crisis in January 2009 that started with vomiting and diarrhea, which made me so weak that I could not walk. The pain in my back and legs was ignored because I had back surgery four months prior. After falling three times, the EMS was called. I went into respiratory arrest before they arrived, but thanks to my partner knowing CPR, I was revived.

The EMS did not apparently did not understand Addison's, and the emergency room also was very slow to react to my needs. Finally after I had total kidney failure and a temp of 104, they put me in ICU to address my crisis. I was in the hospital for eight days.

Two months later, I am now experiencing moderate to severe fatigue. My doctors say that it is not Addison's, but I beg to differ. They think that I am just depressed. I am very frustrated at this point. Is the fatigue due to Addison's?

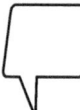

I can attest that Addison's can be associated with severe fatigue, so I agree it's probably associate with your problems.

ADDISON'S DISEASE

Did you recently take an antibiotic? If so it may be related to an intestinal yeast infection. The yeast byproducts are released into your gut and if you are sensitive to those, you can feel great fatigue. Addison's makes it easy for yeast to grow, so it's also important to cut back on all sugar products because those make yeast grow fast.

Zinc, selenium, vitamin D and vitamin C are known to support your immune system and I strongly recommend you start taking those along with a multi-vitamin.

I have been fine since being diagnosed with Addison's diagnosis, living life to the fullest, enjoying it, and everything was peachy... until last weekend. Something seems to have snapped in my head and I do not know what hit me or how to fix it. I have been so sick, not able to eat, not able to handle doing the things I used to do all the time. I am scared, tense and feel like there is someone else in my head that is evil. I have lost weight, have shaking and crying spells, sweating and chills. I did go to my family doctor and talked in depth about this and she feels that it is a combination of things including stress and medication dosage. I am going to talk to her again on Monday but as of right now I would

not say it is getting any better. Has anyone else experienced this and if so what was it and what fixed it?

> This is exactly how I feel before I go into a crisis. Make sure you are getting enough hydrocortisone.

> I also feel like this before I am going into crisis or if I have had a particularly stressful day or week. The shaking and crying happens to me and it's very frustrating. I would work to reduce whatever stressors you have in your life right now and possibly double your medications (particularly your prednisone, if you take that).

ADDISON'S DISEASE

DIAGNOSIS

Suggestive features

Routine investigations may show:[3]

- Hypercalcemia

- Hypoglycemia, low blood sugar (worse in children)

- Hyponatraemia (low blood sodium levels), due to loss of production of the hormone aldosterone

- Hyperkalemia (raised blood potassium levels), also due to loss of production of the hormone aldosterone

- Eosinophilia and lymphocytosis (increased number of eosinophils or lymphocytes, two types of white blood cells)

- Metabolic acidosis (increased blood acidity), also due to loss of the hormone aldosterone because sodium reabsorption in the distal tubule is linked with acid/hydrogen ion (H+) secretion. Low levels of aldosterone stimulation of the renal distal tubule leads to sodium wasting in the urine and H+ retention in the serum.

 *I have just been diagnosed with Addison's this week and was told I have complete adrenal*

failure. My doctor thinks I have more going on than just Addison's disease as well, but my endocrinologist can't see me for at least another eight weeks as he is too busy. I have been told they want me in hospital as soon as possible, but due to the lack of beds and staff, this is not possible at the moment.

Has anyone had to wait this long before seeing their endocrinologist? I was sent home from the hospital with just my medication and no information about the disease at all.

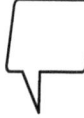

I cannot really address the Addison's issue but I would suggest that you take charge of your own health and get a copy of the test results for yourself. The adrenal glands produce a variety of hormones including testosterone, aldosterone and cortisol. All of these steroids control many things in your body including your blood pressure, how you handle stress, and your gynecological functions such as ovulation, menstruation, etc. There is a large variety of problems that can occur with adrenal glands and sometimes the adrenals simply have a problem converting the precursor of these hormones into the hormones themselves. You may therefore be experiencing an imbalance of these hormones and this would be causing your *problems. The steroids are the treatment of choice at the moment. However, the medication may need to be adjusted or perhaps another type of steroid tried in order to fit your specific situation. All will depend on what your endocrinologist has to say.*

I would also try to find an endocrinologist a little sooner. Ask some of your friends or family if they happen to know anyone or call the association of endocrinologists in your country or area and see if they can suggest something.

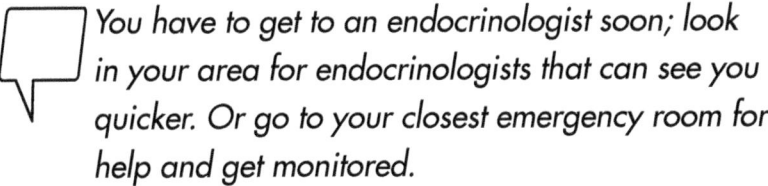 You have to get to an endocrinologist soon; look in your area for endocrinologists that can see you quicker. Or go to your closest emergency room for help and get monitored.

Testing

In suspected cases of Addison's disease, one needs to demonstrate that adrenal hormone levels are low even after appropriate stimulation (called the adrenocorticotropic hormone stimulation test) with synthetic pituitary adrenocorticotropic hormone tetracosactide. Two tests are performed, the short and the long test.

The short test compares blood cortisol levels before and after 250 micrograms of tetracosactide (IM/IV) is given. If, one hour later, plasma cortisol exceeds 170 nmol/L and has risen by at least 330 nmol/L to at least 690 nmol/L, adrenal failure is excluded. If the short test is abnormal, the long test is used to differentiate between primary adrenal failure and secondary adrenocortical failure.

The long test uses 1 mg tetracosactide (IM). Blood is taken 1, 4, 8, and 24 hours later. Normal plasma cortisol level should reach 1000 nmol/L by four hours. In primary Addison's disease, the cortisol level is reduced at all stages whereas in secondary corticoadrenal insufficiency, a delayed but normal response is seen.

Other tests that may be performed to distinguish between various causes of hypoadrenalism are renin and adrenocorticotropic hormone levels, as well as medical imaging - usually in the form of ultrasound, computed tomography or magnetic resonance imaging (MRI).

Adrenoleukodystrophy, and the milder form, adrenomyeloneuropathy, cause adrenal insufficiency combined with neurological symptoms. These diseases are estimated to be the cause of adrenal insufficiency in approximately 35% of male patients with idiopathic Addison's disease and should be

ADDISON'S DISEASE

considered in the differential diagnosis of any male with adrenal insufficiency. Diagnosis is made by a blood test to detect very long chain fatty acids (VLCFA).[7]

I was wondering if anyone here has been diagnosed with secondary or tertiary Addison's? My primary physician is convinced that this is what has been plaguing me for almost five years now. She referred me to an Endocrinologist, and I see him this afternoon. I only have my lab results from 2005, which are:

AM Cortisol- 8.6 & 8.2 (ref range 6–22, taken one week apart)

adrenocorticotropic hormone 10 (ref range 10–60)

While Addison's disease certainly fits the profile of my symptoms, my labs were still within the normal range. I am wondering why they suspect Addison's.

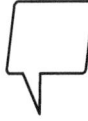

The lab scales are for normal people with no symptoms. If you are experiencing symptoms of low cortisol and you have low end test results, then it's reasonable to at least test to rule out cortisol problems. Low cortisol AND low

adrenocorticotropic hormone at the same time is also a good indicator of trouble.

A blood test is not diagnostic; instead you need some kind of provocative test that determines your actual adrenal capacity. If you were to be seriously stressed with low cortisol, you could be in a deadly situation. Undiscovered low cortisol kills several people each year.

CAUSES

Causes of adrenal insufficiency can be grouped by the way in which they cause the adrenals to produce insufficient cortisol. These are adrenal dysgenesis (the gland has not formed adequately during development), impaired steroidogenesis (the gland is present but is biochemically unable to produce cortisol) or adrenal destruction (disease processes leading to the gland being damaged).[3]

Adrenal dysgenesis

All causes in this category are genetic, and generally very rare. These include mutations to the SF1 transcription factor, congenital adrenal hypoplasia (AHC) due to DAX-1 gene mutations and mutations to the adrenocorticotropic hormone receptor gene (or related genes, such as in the Triple A or Allgrove syndrome). DAX-1 mutations may cluster in a syndrome with glycerol kinase deficiency with a number of other symptoms when DAX-1 is deleted together with a number of other genes.[3]

Impaired steroidogenesis

To form cortisol, the adrenal gland requires cholesterol, which is then converted biochemically into steroid hormones. Interruptions in the delivery of cholesterol include Smith-Lemli-Opitz syndrome and abetalipoproteinemia.

Of the synthesis problems, congenital adrenal hyperplasia is the most common (in various forms: 21-hydroxylase, 17α-hydroxylase, 11β-hydroxylase and 3β-hydroxysteroid dehydrogenase), lipod CAH due to deficiency of StAR and mitochondrial DNA mutations.[3] Some medications interfere with steroid synthesis enzymes (e.g. ketoconazole), while others accelerate the normal breakdown of hormones by the liver (e.g. rifampicin, phenytoin).[3]

Adrenal destruction

Autoimmune adrenalitis can be a cause of Addison's disease. Autoimmune destruction of the adrenal cortex (often due to antibodies against the enzyme 21-Hydroxylase) is a common cause of Addison's in teenagers and adults. This may be isolated or in the context of autoimmune polyendocrine syndrome (APS type 1 or 2).

Adrenal destruction is also a feature of adrenoleukodystrophy (ALD), and when the adrenal glands are involved in metastasis (seeding of cancer cells from elsewhere in the body, especially lung), hemorrhage (e.g. in Waterhouse-Friderichsen syndrome or antiphospholipid syndrome), particular infections (tuberculosis,[8] histoplasmosis, coccidioidomycosis), deposition of abnormal protein in amyloidosis.

HEALTHSCOUTER

ADDISON'S DISEASE

TREATMENT

Maintenance treatment

Treatment for Addison's disease involves replacing the missing cortisol, usually in the form of hydrocortisone tablets, in a dosing regimen that mimics the physiological concentrations of cortisol. Alternatively one quarter as much prednisolone may be used for equal glucocorticoid effect as hydrocortisone. Treatment must usually be continued for life. In addition, many patients require fludrocortisone as replacement for the missing aldosterone. Caution must be exercised when the person with Addison's disease becomes unwell, has surgery or becomes pregnant. Medication may need to be increased during times of stress, infection, or injury.

My daughter was diagnosed with Addison's. Do you think she will gain a lot of weight with being on the steroids?

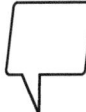

If your daughter is on the proper replacement dose, she should not gain a lot of weight. However, now that she is on medication she will gain some or all of the weight she lost before diagnosis. The

key is to find the correct dose to help her function normally.

EPIDEMIOLOGY

The frequency rate of Addison's disease in the human population is sometimes estimated at roughly one in 100,000.[9] Some research and information sites put the number closer to 40–60 cases per 1 million population. (1/25,000-1/16,600)[10] (Determining accurate numbers for Addison's is problematic at best and some incidence figures are thought to be underestimates.[11]) Addison's can afflict persons of any age, gender, or ethnicity, but it typically presents in adults between 30 and 50 years of age.[12] Research has shown no significant predispositions based on ethnicity.[10]

ADDISON'S DISEASE

PROGNOSIS

With proper medication, patients can expect to live a healthy and normal life.

I have been seeing a girl who was diagnosed with Addison's when she was 13. She is 21 now and told me recently that she is not having trouble with the symptoms of Addison's; it's the dealing with the treatments/medication/doctors/specialists everyday that she is tired of. She also sees little hope for the future because she does not expect to have a long and healthy life because she is living with an incurable disease.

I want to help her so that she can feel as though her condition isn't controlling her life. It's hard to provide encouragement to someone when you are not in the same position as they are and do not fully understand the challenges they face every day because I have not faced them.

I need to know how I can help someone with the non-medical side of Addison's. Dealing with and handling stressful conditions, depression, fatigue, etc. What would you want your mate/partner to do when you are not feeling so hot about your life and the way you have to live it? Is there anything specifically that would make you feel better?

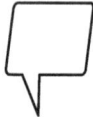
President Kennedy had Addison's, and he certainly lived a very normal, active life. If he can do it in a time when they knew little about this disease, then your new girlfriend can also.

While it might be true that Addison's is not curable, there is a lot of hope for the future regarding treatments, including injectable spheres that slowly dissolve and provide a month's worth of cortisol at a time.

The main problem with Addison's is when other problems compound the situation. If your girlfriend is not feeling well then that means something is still amiss. Perhaps she should try taking DHEA. Perhaps she still has an intestinal yeast problem, which was caused by years of low cortisol. Perhaps she has other health problems unrelated to Addison's, such as low thyroid, or other pituitary hormone deficiencies.

If she is not feeling well then it's time to encourage her to see a doctor and get to the bottom of why she isn't feeling normal; because she should be. Addison's is a very livable disease.

ADDISON'S DISEASE

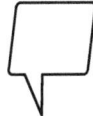 If she isn't feeling well then she needs to find out why. I would suggest a full physical with blood testing of levels such as vitamins, dhea, thyroid, hormones etc. I have been diagnosed for a little over two years now and I feel more normal than I have in more years that I can count. My medications are doing the job and I have a very happy and full life.

HEALTHSCOUTER

ADDISON'S DISEASE

CANINE HYPOADRENOCORTICISM

The condition is relatively rare, but has been diagnosed in all breeds of dogs. In general, it is underdiagnosed, and one has to have a clinical suspicion of it as an underlying disorder for many presenting complaints. Females are overrepresented, and the disease often appears in middle age (4–7 years), although any age or gender may be affected. Genetic continuity between dogs and humans helps to explain the occurrence of Addison's disease in both species.[13]

Hypoadrenocorticism is treated with prednisolone and/or fludrocortisone (Florinef (r)) or a monthly injection called Percorten V (desoxycorticosterone pivlate (DOCP)). Routine blood work is necessary periodically to assess therapy.

Most of the medications used in the therapy of hypoadrenocorticism cause excessive thirst and urination. It is absolutely vital to provide fresh drinking water for the canine sufferer.

If the owner knows about an upcoming stressful situation (shows, traveling etc.), patients generally need an increased dose of prednisone to help deal with the added stress. Avoidance of stress is important for dogs with hypoadrenocorticism.

ADDISON'S DISEASE

ADRENAL INSUFFICIENCY

Adrenal insufficiency is a condition in which the adrenal glands, located above the kidneys, do not produce adequate amounts of steroid hormones (chemicals produced by the body that regulate organ function), primarily cortisol, but may also include impaired aldosterone production (a mineralcorticoid) which regulates sodium, potassium and water retention.[1][2] Craving for salt or salty foods due to the urinary losses of sodium is common.[3]

Addison's disease is the worst degree of adrenal insufficiency, which if not treated, results in severe abdominal pains, diarrhea, vomiting, profound muscle weakness and fatigue, extremely low blood pressure, weight loss, kidney failure, changes in mood and personality and shock may occur (adrenal crisis).[4] An adrenal crisis often occurs if the body is subjected to stress, such as an accident, injury, surgery, or severe infection; death may quickly follow.[4]

Adrenal insufficiency can also occur when the hypothalamus or the pituitary gland, both located at the base of the skull, doesn't make adequate amounts of the hormones that assist in regulating adrenal function.[1][5][6] This is called secondary adrenal insufficiency and is caused by lack of production of adrenocorticotropic hormone in the pituitary or lack of corticotropin releasing hormone in the hypothalamus.[7]

My question in a nutshell is: Can you have both Addison's disease AND secondary adrenal insufficiency?

Basically my adrenocorticotropic hormone was very low, but my cortisol stimulation test also didn't quite double, so I don't understand. I don't meet with my doctor again until Friday. I was hoping to just do some research ahead of time to know what I might be dealing with and what questions to ask.

Also, she has me on hydrocortisone 10 mg in the morning and 5 mg in the evening, but I'm still getting really lightheaded to where sometimes I have to lay down. I do have a home blood pressure monitor and have been getting readings anywhere from 94/60 to 115/75, usually around 110/70. That doesn't seem TOO low, does it? Could the hydrocortisone itself be causing me to be lightheaded or does it sound like I should be on more (the on-call doctor had put me on double that dose but my regular

ADDISON'S DISEASE

endocrinologist called back and said to cut it in half--I felt better on the double dose)?

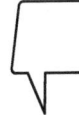I am sorry that you are feeling poorly. But rest assured you cannot have both Addison's and adrenal insufficiency. Adrenal Insufficiency is called secondary Addison's, which means your problem is not autoimmune, which is good. Both diseases are treated with the same medications, and primary Addison's can develop later in life so they keep a monitor on it with antibody tests and by monitoring your cortisol. If they told you to cut back your dose, you are getting too much replacement which is as serious as not enough. You will feel poorly when taking less medication at first but you will adjust.

If you are still light headed and having symptoms, have them continue to run tests.

Types

There are two major types of adrenal insufficiency.

- Primary adrenal insufficiency is due to impairment of the adrenal glands.
  - The most common subtype is called idiopathic or unknown cause of adrenal insufficiency.

- Some are due to an autoimmune disease called Addison's disease or autoimmune adrenalitis.

- Other cases are due to congenital adrenal hyperplasia or an adenoma (tumor) of the adrenal gland.

- Secondary adrenal insufficiency is caused by impairment of the pituitary gland or hypothalamus.[8] These can be due to a form of cancer: a pituitary microadenoma, a pituitary macroadenoma, or a hypothalamic tumor; Sheehan's syndrome, which is associated with impairment of only the pituitary gland; or a past head injury.

My symptoms are: severe fatigue, nausea, blacking out when standing up, low blood pressure (90/55), lower back pain, change in my skin tone to coppery, unable to recover after exercise or any stressful event, weird headaches. And I also lost over 10 pounds. I had the adrenocorticotropic hormone stimulation test done, between 10–11am and the results were:

Baseline cortison: 449 nmol/L (16.27 ug/dl)

After 60 minutes: 491 nmol/L (17.79 ug/dl)

ADDISON'S DISEASE

To me, these results do suggest some form of adrenal insufficiency; they obviously do not respond well to stimulation by adrenocorticotropic hormone.

 Your symptoms sound like Addison's disease. Go see a specialist.

Causes

- Autoimmune - may be part of a polyglandular autoimmune disorder which can include type I Diabetes Mellitus, autoimmune thyroid disease (also known as autoimmune thyroiditis, Hashimoto's thyroiditis and Hashimoto's disease)[9]

- Adrenoleukodystrophy[10]

- Discontinuing corticosteroid therapy without tapering the dosage (severe adrenal suppression with adrenocorticotropic hormone suppression)

- Illness or any other forms of stress (this is termed critical illness–related corticosteroid insufficiency)

- Kidney injury

- Environmental

- Genetics

- Head injury

- Radiation
- Surgery
- Infections (e.g., miliary tuberculosis affecting the adrenal glands, meningitis)
- Congenital hypopituitarism
- Congential hypoadrenalism

Symptoms

The person may show symptoms of hypoglycemia, dehydration, weight loss and disorientation. They may experience weakness, tiredness, dizziness, low blood pressure that falls further when standing (orthostatic hypotension), muscle aches, nausea, vomiting, and diarrhea. These problems may develop gradually and insidiously. Addison's can present with tanning of the skin which may be patchy or even all over the body. In some cases a person with normally light skin may be mistaken for another race with darker pigmentation. Characteristic sites of tanning are skin creases (e.g. of the hands) and the inside of the cheek (buccal mucosa). Goitre and vitiligo may also be present.[4]

I am hypothyroid. I am 44 years old. Since October I have been in a brain fog, basal temp

ADDISON'S DISEASE

of 95.2–95.5, nausea, extreme dizziness, chest pain, knee pain, heart palpitations, horrible headaches, huge lump in my throat feeling, extremely dry skin, hair falling out, horrible anxiety, and I was told my hormone levels show that I am almost done with perimenopause, that they are extremely low for my age. Everyone wants to tell me it is just stress and to deal with it. I have never felt so horrible in all my life. There have been many days that I cannot even get out of my bed. I am on 100mcg synthroid. It worked for me for years but now when I take it some days my heart starts racing and I get an abnormal heart rhythm and panic attacks, other days I feel nothing and I am so dead tired and physically sick that I can't stand it. Has anyone else ever felt so bad?

Your symptoms sound very similar to what my daughter was experiencing before she was diagnosed with adrenal insufficiency. Have you seen an endocrinologist? Low blood pressure was her primary symptom, although she did have headaches and heart palpitations, too. She was sent to an endocrinologist for further testing and she got her diagnosis.

Diagnosis

If the person is in adrenal crisis, the adrenocorticotropic hormone stimulation test may be given. If not in crisis, cortisol, adrenocorticotropic hormone, aldosterone, renin, potassium and sodium are tested from a blood sample before the decision is made if the adrenocorticotropic hormone stimulation test needs to be performed. X-rays or CT of the adrenals may also be done.[1] The best test for adrenal insufficiency of autoimmune origin, representing more than 90% of all cases in a Western population, is measurement of 21-hydroxylase autoantibodies (Winqvist O, Karlsson FA, Kampe O, Lancet 1992).

Treatment

- Adrenal crisis
    - Intravenous fluids[4]
    - Intravenous steroid (Solu-Cortef or Solumedrol), later hydrocortisone, prednisone or methylpredisolone tablets[4]
        - Rest
- Cortisol deficiency (primary and secondary)

ADDISON'S DISEASE

- Adrenal cortical extract (usually in the form of a supplement, non prescription in the United States)

- Hydrocortisone (Cortef) (between 20 and 35 mg)[4]

- Prednisone (Deltasone) (7 1/2 mg)

- Prednisolone (Delta-Cortef) (7 1/2 mg)

- Methylprednisolone (Medrol) (6 mg)

- Dexamethasone (Decadron) (1/4 mg, some doctors prescribe 1/2 to 1 mg, but those doses tend to cause side effects resembling Cushing's disease)

- Mineralcorticoid deficiency (low aldosterone)

  - Fludrocortisone (Florinef) (To balance sodium, potassium and increase water retention)[4]

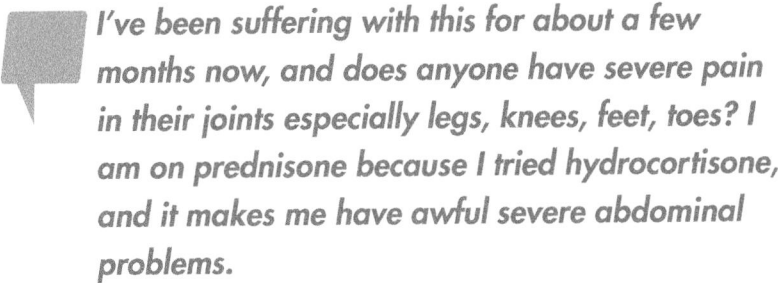

I've been suffering with this for about a few months now, and does anyone have severe pain in their joints especially legs, knees, feet, toes? I am on prednisone because I tried hydrocortisone, and it makes me have awful severe abdominal problems.

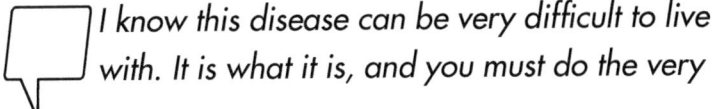

I know this disease can be very difficult to live with. It is what it is, and you must do the very

best you can to manage it. I do not believe that the prednisone is the cause of your physical pain. In fact, prednisone is often prescribed for pain/inflammation throughout the body. Physical pain/inflammation is often due to LOW cortisol levels. My gut tells me that you're not taking enough cortisol.

I have recently switched to prednisone from hydrocortisone. Prednisone works better for me because it is a longer acting steroid so I don't have to take it as often as I was taking the hydrocortisone.

ADRENOCORTICOTROPIC HORMONE STIMULATION TEST

The adrenocorticotropic hormone stimulation test (also called the *cosyntropin test* or *tetracosactide test*) is a medical test usually ordered and interpreted by endocrinologists to assess the functioning of the adrenal glands stress response by measuring the adrenal response to adrenocorticotropic hormone (ACTH).[1][2] adrenocorticotropic hormone is a hormone produced in the pituitary gland that stimulates the adrenal glands to release cortisol.[2]

During the test, a small amount of synthetic adrenocorticotropic hormone is injected, and the amount of cortisol, and sometimes aldosterone, the adrenals produce in response is measured.[3] This test may cause mild to moderate side effects in some individuals.[4][5]

This test is used to diagnose or exclude primary and secondary adrenal insufficiency, Addison's disease and related conditions.[2] In addition to quantifying adrenal insufficiency, the test can distinguish whether the cause is adrenal (low cortisol and aldosterone production) or pituitary (low adrenocorticotropic hormone production).[1] The adrenocorticotropic hormone stimulation test is recognized by the medical community as the final say in whether or not an individual has a degree of adrenal insufficiency, although this test is primarily used to determine the presence of Addison's disease and pituitary impairment.[6] If the test does not show Addison's, the test interpreter may see it as showing the adrenal glands are working, not recognizing any degree of adrenal insufficiency between Addison's (the worst degree of adrenal insufficiency) and healthy adrenal function. Secondary adrenal insufficiency is often overlooked by uninformed interpreters of this test.

Adrenal insufficiency is a potentially life-threatening condition. Treatment should be initiated as soon as the diagnosis is confirmed, or sooner if the patient presents in adrenal crisis

I am forty years old, and have been in a lot of pain starting over 10 years back. This past year, they told me I probably have Fibromyalgia, but I discovered Addison's a few weeks back. I am being tested to see if that is what I actually have this week. Has anybody had anything similar happen to them?

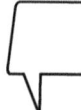
I am 38, and for years I was told that I had chronic fatigue syndrome and "to just live with it!" In May this year I had what is called an Addisonian crisis.

My blood pressure dropped to 80/50 at the time of admitting to the hospital and when the team of six doctors that were working tirelessly on me through the night to ensure that I lived through it brought in an endocrinologist, he immediately ran the ACHT blood test. When it came back it was conclusive and the diagnosis was also conclusive - I do indeed have Addison's disease. The BEST choice to seek for Addison's disease would be an endocrinologist (or hematologist) - they are knowledgeable in the disease and know how to treat and diagnose.

Versions of the test

This test can be given as a *low-dose short test*, a *conventional-dose short test*, or as a *prolonged-stimulation test*.

In the low-dose short test, 1 microgram of an adrenocorticotropic hormone drug is injected into the patient. In the conventional-dose short test, 250 μg of drug are injected. Both of these short tests last for about an hour and provide the same information. Studies have shown the measured stress response of the adrenals is the same for the low-dose and conventional-dose tests.[8]

The prolonged-stimulation test, which is also called a *long conventional-dose test,* can last up to 48 hours. This form of the test can differentiate between primary, secondary, and tertiary adrenal insufficiency. This form of the test is rarely performed because earlier testing of cortisol and adrenocorticotropic hormone levels in association with the short test may provide all the necessary information.[7]

I have been struggling with hypoglycemia and low blood pressures along with a host of other stuff. Recently my blood pressure had been dropping even lower and has begun to concern me. This past morning I could barely get up and was very confused. I couldn't remember where I was or what was going on. My blood pressure was 63/47 once I became coherent enough to check it. I have come to the conclusion I better get tested for Addison's. I need to know exactly what tests I should ask my doctor to do as I can't afford to waste money on any unnecessary tests.

Also, if this truly is my problem and I get started on steroids, how long will it take to make me stronger again?

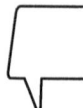

Ask your doctor to order the adrenocorticotropic hormone stimulation test and ensure it is done first

thing in the morning by a laboratory that knows what it is doing. It can be a tricky test if not done correctly. Your doctor can also do a baseline, random Coritsol, but I trust this less, because what the body produces goes through such a pendulum swing that the 'results' have a wide range of normal.

If you aren't aware, the adrenocorticotropic hormone stimulation test tests a baseline cortisol first, then they inject you with a precursor hormone which stimulates the adrenal glands to respond. They then draw your blood 30, 60, and 90 minutes after the IV injection to see if your adrenals truly did respond. This test is the best diagnostic tool for Adrenal Insufficiency that I know of.

And as for how long you will be feeling better, that depends! Some people feel better right away when they start the steroids, like magic! I felt progressively better; it took me three years to feel as good as I do right now, and right now I feel pretty great!

Preparation

The person must fast at least eight hours before the test which should be started by 10 am, but as close to 7 am as possible.[9] The test shouldn't be given if on glucocorticoids, pregnenolone, or adrenal extract supplement as these will affect test results. Stress and recently administered radioisotope scans can artificially increase levels and may invalidate test results. Spironolactone, contraceptives, licorice, estrogen, androgen (including DHEA) and progesterone therapy may also affect both aldosterone and cortisol stimulation test results.[10][11] If aldosterone is to be stimulated, salt and foods significant in sodium must be fasted for 24 hours prior to testing. This allows aldosterone to rise as far as possible. Women must test the first week of their cycle or aldosterone (and occasionally cortisol) results may appear ok in the last half of the cycle when progesterone is higher (progesterone breaks down into aldosterone and cortisol).[12]

Administration

Blood is drawn to get a starting or base cortisol (adrenocorticotropic hormone is also tested from this draw) and or aldosterone level. Next, synthetic adrenocorticotropic hormone (Synacthen aka Tetracosactide or Cortrosyn aka Cosyntropin) is injected. Approximately 20 mL of heparinized venous blood is collected at 30 and 60 minutes after the synthetic adrenocorticotropic hormone injection.[13][14]

All blood samples are kept on ice and sent immediately to the laboratory for testing.[9]

I just had an Adrenocorticotropic Hormone Stimulation Test yesterday and would like your opinions on the results. I thought for sure I had Addison's, have all the symptoms except for the hyperpigmentation. Now I'm leaning more towards secondary.

I had a Cortisol test back on July 17th. The draw at 8AM showed that my reading was 6.0 ug/dl (reference range 4–23).

Adrenocorticotropic Hormone Stimulation Test my endocrinologist ordered showed:

Base level drawn at 7:55AM, fasting was 9.8 ug/dl

30 minute draw was 21.6 ug/dl

60 minute draw was 24.8 ug/dl

From these results does anyone have anything to share with me?

You had a noticeable cortisol response and both numbers were within the normal range. Most likely

your endocrinologist will think the adrenals are functioning.

However, it does not rule out a pituitary origin for the adrenal problems and that will have to be investigated with an insulin induced hypoglycemia test.

Potential side effects

Normal reactions that should be reported are nausea, anxiety, sweating, dizziness, itchy skin, redness and or swelling of injection site, palpitations (a fast or fluttering heart beat) and facial flushing (may also include arms and torso), but should disappear within a few hours.[4][5] Rarely seen, but serious side effects include rash, fainting, headache, blurred vision, severe swelling, severe dizziness, trouble breathing, irregular heartbeat.[5]

Although uncommon, some people report feeling better or sense of well being after the test.

Interpretation of results

Cortisol stimulation

In healthy individuals, the cortisol level should double from a value at least in the 20s within 60 minutes.

If the cortisol level was a 25 before the stimulation (base level), after the stimulation it should reach at least 50 ug/dl.

Interpretation for primary adrenal insufficiency and Addison's disease

The base cortisol level in people with adrenal insufficiency is usually in the mid teens. If the adrenocorticotropic hormone stimulation test raises cortisol level to 20 ug/dl, that is not doubling and supports the diagnosis of primary adrenal insufficiency. In Addison's, base cortisol is well below 10 ug/dl and rises no more than 25 percent.

Interpretation for secondary adrenal insufficiency

Adrenocorticotropic hormone may stimulate cortisol by a factor doubling, tripling, quadrupling or more from a low base value in patients suffering from secondary adrenal insufficiency. Stimulation resulting in a greater than 14-fold increase in serum concentration over 30 minutes has been reported; however in most cases serum cortisol levels only double or triple and most start with a base cortisol value of at least 10 ug/dl. The lower the base cortisol value, the more likely the patient's cortisol will stimulate by a high factor if they are secondary adrenal insufficient.[9]

In some instances, a second test performed later can suggest primary adrenal insufficiency (cortisol value less than doubled). The diagnosis may be changed from secondary to primary adrenal insufficiency or to include primary adrenal insufficiency. In secondary adrenal insufficiency, if the adrenal glands lack adrenocorticotropic hormone for enough time, cortisol production can atrophy[15] and fail to rise to a value at least double the base cortisol value. It is proper to continue with the diagnosis of secondary adrenal insufficiency.

If secondary adrenal insufficiency is diagnosed, the insulin tolerance test (ITT) or the CRH (Corticotropin-releasing hormone) stimulation test can be used to distinguish between a hypothalamic (tertiary) and pituitary (secondary) cause, but is rarely used in clinical practice.[15]

Adrenocorticotropic hormone plasma test plus cortisol stimulation

An adrenocorticotropic hormone plasma test should always be given at the same time as the adrenocorticotropic hormone stimulation, although many doctors consider the test inaccurate. This test measures how much adrenocorticotropic hormone the pituitary gland is producing. A healthy

ADDISON'S DISEASE

adrenocorticotropic hormone value should be just into the upper third of the range (assuming a range of 10–60 ng/L). The adrenocorticotropic hormone plasma and adrenocorticotropic hormone stimulation test together can give a clearer picture, especially for secondary adrenal insufficiency.[13]

Interpretation for primary adrenal insufficiency and Addison's disease

adrenocorticotropic hormone will be high[13] - either at the top or above range. In Addison's disease, adrenocorticotropic hormone may be way above range and may reach the hundreds. In very rare cases can reach the 1000s and 2000s.

Interpretation for secondary adrenal insufficiency

Adrenocorticotropic hormone will be low[13] - Usually below 35, but most people with secondary fall within the range limit. Although uncommon, values for adrenocorticotropic hormone can reach into the low 40s.

In some cases, actual cause of low adrenocorticotropic hormone is from low corticotropin releasing hormone in the hypothalamus. It is possible to have separate adrenocorticotropic hormone and corticotropin releasing hormone impairment such as can happen in a head injury.[16]

Aldosterone stimulation

The adrenocorticotropic hormone stimulation test is occasionally used to test adrenal production of aldosterone at the same time as cortisol to also help in determining if primary (hyperreninemic) or secondary (hyporeninemic) hypoaldosteronism is present.[3] Human adrenocorticotropic hormone has a slight stimulatory effect on aldosterone[17], but the amount of synthetic adrenocorticotropic hormone given in the stimulation is equivalent to more than a whole days production of natural adrenocorticotropic hormone, so the aldosterone response can be easily measured in blood serum.[18] Same as cortisol, aldosterone should double from a respectable base value (around 20 ng/dl, must fast salt 24 hours and sit upright for blood draw) in a healthy individual.

Interpretation for primary aldosterone deficiency

The aldosterone response in the adrenocorticotropic hormone stimulation test is blunted or absent in patients with primary adrenal insufficiency including Addison's disease.[3] The base value is usually in the mid teens or less and rise to less than double the base value thus indicating primary hypoaldosteronism (sodium low, potassium and renin enzyme will be high) and is an indicator of primary adrenal insufficiency or Addison's disease.

Interpretation for secondary aldosterone deficiency

Aldosterone response of several factors from a low base value. This factoring indicates secondary hypoaldosteronism (sodium low, potassium and renin enzyme will be low). Usually doubling to quadrupling from a low base aldosterone value is what is seen in secondary adrenal insufficiency. Decupling of aldosterone in the adrenocorticotropic hormone stimulation test is possible (i.e. 2 ng/dl stimming to 20).[19] A result of doubling of more of aldosterone may help in tandem with a cortisol stimulation that doubled or more confirm a diagnosis of secondary adrenal insufficiency. In rare cases, an aldosterone stimulation which did not double, but with the presence of low potassium, low renin and low adrenocorticotropic hormone indicates atrophy of aldosterone production from the prolonged lack of renin.

Similar to the cortisol stimulation in adrenocorticotropic hormone deficiency, the test interpreter may lack knowledge of how to properly interpret for secondary hypoaldosteronism and think a result of aldosterone doubling or more from a low base value is good.

Other hormones and chemicals that will rise in the adrenocorticotropic hormone stimulation test

- Progesterone - precursor to cortisol and aldosterone[20]

- Luteinizing hormone - a pituitary hormone that stimulates sex hormone production[20]

- 21-Hydroxylase[21]

- DHEA and DHEA-S (an androgen hormone produced in the adrenal glands)

ADRENOLEUKODYSTROPHY

Adrenoleukodystrophy (ALD) (also known as "Addison-Schilder Disease," "Siemerling-Creutzfeldt Disease," and "Schilder's disease"[1]:545) is a rare, inherited disorder that leads to progressive brain damage, failure of the adrenal glands and eventually death. adrenoleukodystrophy is one disease in a group of inherited disorders called leukodystrophies. Adrenoleukodystrophy progressively damages the myelin, a complex fatty neural tissue that insulates many nerves of the central and peripheral nervous systems, eventually destroying it. Without myelin, nerves are unable to conduct an impulse, leading to increasing disability as myelin destruction increases and intensifies.

An essential protein, called a transporter protein, is missing in sufferers. This protein is needed to carry an enzyme which is used to break down very long-chain fatty acids found in the normal diet. Lack of this protein can give rise to a build-up of very long-chain fatty acids, (VLCFA) in the body which can damage the brain and the adrenal gland.

There are several different types of the disease which can be inherited, but the most common form is an X-linked condition. Patients with X-linked adrenoleukodystrophy are all male, but about one in five women carrying the disease develop some symptoms. *Adrenomyeloneuropathy* is a less-severe form of adrenoleukodystrophy, with onset of symptoms occurring in adolescence or adulthood. This milder form does not include cerebral involvement, and should be included in the differential diagnosis of all males with adrenal insufficiency.

Although this disorder affects the growth and/or development of myelin, leukodystrophies are different from demyelinating disorders such as multiple sclerosis where myelin is formed normally but is lost by immunologic dysfunction or for other reasons.

Symptoms

The clinical presentation is largely dependent on the age of onset of the disease. The classical, severe type is the childhood cerebral form which, as an X-linked disease, affects males. Symptoms normally start between the ages of four and 10 and include loss of previously acquired neurologic abilities, seizures, ataxia, Addison's disease, as well as degeneration of visual and auditory function. It has been seen that infants that have been positively diagnosed by the age of one year old have usually become very ill by the age of 10 to 12 years of age and die soon after. This severe form of the disease was first described by Ernst Siemerling and Hans Gerhard Creutzfeldt.[2] A similar form can also occur in adolescents and very rarely in adults. Addison's disease can be an initial symptom of adrenoleukodystrophy, and many pediatric endocrinologists will measure very long chain free fatty acids in newly diagnosed males with this condition, as a screening test for adrenoleukodystrophy.

In another form of adrenoleukodystrophy which primarily strikes young men, the spinal cord dysfunction is more prominent and therefore is called *adrenomyeloneuropathy*, or "AMN." The patients usually present with weakness and numbness of the limbs and urination or defecation problems. Most victims of this form are also males, although some female carriers exhibit symptoms of adrenomyeloneuropathy.[3]

Adult and neonatal forms of the disease also exist but they are extremely rare. (These tend to affect both males and females and be inherited in an autosomal recessive manner.) Some patients may present with sole findings of adrenal insufficiency.

adrenoleukodystrophy also causes uncontrollable rage in some cases.

Diagnosis

The diagnosis is established by clinical findings and the detection of serum very long-chain free fatty acid levels.[4] MRI examination reveals white matter abnormalities, and neuro-imaging findings of this disease are somewhat reminiscent of the findings of multiple sclerosis. Genetic testing for the analysis of the defective gene is available in some centers.

Neonatal screening may become available in the future, which may permit early diagnosis and treatment.[5] Approximately one in 42,000 boys are diagnosed with X-linked adrenoleukodystrophy.[6]

Pathophysiology

X-linked

The most common form of adrenoleukodystrophy is X-linked, which means that the defective gene is on the X chromosome. It is located at Xq28, and the disease is characterized by excessive accumulation of very long-chain fatty acids (VLCFA), which are fatty acids with chains of 24–30 carbon atoms. The most common is hexacosanoate, with a 26 carbon skeleton.

The elevation in (VLCFA) was originally described by Moser *et al.* in 1981.[7] The adrenoleukodystrophy gene was discovered in 1993, and it coded for a protein that was a member of a family of transporter proteins, not an enzyme. It is unknown how high levels of very long chain fatty acids cause the loss of myelin.

The gene (ABCD1 or "ATP-binding cassette, subfamily D, member 1") codes for a protein that transfers fatty acids into peroxisomes, the cellular organelles where the fatty acids undergo β-oxidation.[8] A dysfunctional gene leads to the accumulation of very long chain fatty acids (VLCFA). The precise mechanisms through which high VLCFA concentrations cause the disease were still unknown as of 2005, but they do accumulate in the organs affected.

The incidence of X-linked adrenoleukodystrophy is at least one in 42,000 male births.[9]

Autosomal

Autosomal adrenoleukodystrophy has been associated with PEX1, PEX5, PEX10, PEX13, and PEX26.[10]

Treatment

While there is currently no cure for the disease, some dietary treatments, for example, a 4:1 mixture of glyceryl trioleate and glyceryl trierucate (Lorenzo's oil) in combination with a diet low in VLCSFA (very long chain of saturated fatty acids), have been used with limited success, especially before disease symptoms appear. A 2005 study shows positive long-term results with this approach.[11] A 2007 report also appraises "Lorenzo's oil".[12] See also the Myelin Project. X-linked adrenoleukodystrophy has a very variable clinical course, even within a single family.[13] It is therefore not possible to determine if Lorenzo's oil is preventing progression of the disease in asymptomatic patients, or if these patients would have remained asymptomatic even without treatment. Current double blind placebo-controlled trials may be able to answer the questions regarding the effectiveness of treatment.

Hematopoietic stem cell transplantation (HSCT, including bone marrow transplant) is thought to be able to stop the progression of the disease in asymptomatic or mildly symptomatic boys who have a Loes score lower than 9 (an MRI measure of the severity of the disease), though outcomes are markedly poorer in symptomatic boys.[14]

Hematopoietic stem cell transplantation carries a risk of mortality and morbidity and is not recommended for patients whose symptoms are already severe. Umbilical cord blood stem cell transplant may provide an alternative for patients who do not have a matched related stem cell donor. Preliminary studies suggest that the outcome of cord blood stem cell transplant for adrenoleukodystrophy is particularly good in very young, presymptomatic patients.[15]

Lovastatin is an anti-cholesterol drug that appears to have some effect *in vitro*, but not in mice with the animal model of adrenoleukodystrophy.[16] A clinical study of lovastatin showed encouraging biochemical changes, but no objective clinical improvement.[17] Currently, researchers at The Children's Hospital at the University of Minnesota, Dr. Charnas and Dr. Orchard, are investigating Mucomyst as an adjunct to bone marrow transplant, with some increase in survival time after transplant in three patients.[18]

According to a 1986 study, Oleic acid may lower the levels of very long chain free fatty acids in vitro.[19]

Prognosis

Treatment is symptomatic. Progressive neurological degeneration makes the prognosis generally poor. Death occurs within one to ten years of presentation of symptoms. The use of Lorenzo's Oil or of bone marrow transplant are currently under investigation.

Research

Active clinical trials are currently in progress to see if proposed treatments are effective or not:[20]

- Glyceryl Trioleate (Lorenzo's oil) for Adrenomyelneuropathy.[21]

- Beta Interferon and Thalidomide[22] This study is closed.

- Combination of Glyceryl Trierucate and Glyceryl Trioleate (Lorenzo's Oil) in assymptomatic patients.[23]

- Hematopoietic stem cell transplantation[24]

ADRENOMYELONEUROPATHY

Adrenomyeloneuropathy (AMN) is a rare inherited disorder. It is a milder form of X-linked adrenoleukodystrophy (X-adrenoleukodystrophy). In adrenoleukodystrophy, young children generally exhibit cerebral dysfunction, with rapid progression to dementia and quadriparesis. Adrenomyeloneuropathy progresses more slowly, with patients first showing symptoms of weakness and spasticity in adolescence or adulthood. Patients also develop adrenal insufficiency, (Addison's Disease). The gene responsible is located on the long arm of chromosome X, resulting in a sex linked pattern of expression. Males carrying any of several mutations in the gene (known as hemizygous) will always be affected, with about 50% developing X-adrenoleukodystrophy in early childhood and about 50% developing adrenomyeloneuropathy as adolescents or adults. It is unknown why there is such a range in severity of expression, but forms of the disease are found in within the same affected families, (same mutation).[1] The various forms of the disease affect one in 21,000 males.[2]

This disease is caused by defective beta-oxidation of fatty acids in peroxisomes that leads to elevated serum concentrations of very-long-chain saturated fatty acids (VLCFA) and accumulation of cholesterol esters of the fatty acids and gangliosides in the membranes of cells in the brain, adrenal cortex, and other organs. In adrenomyeloneuropathy, this accumulation causes a primary adrenal insufficiency and progressive neurological dysfunction.

Presentation

Adrenomyeloneuropathy begins in adolescence or adulthood. The mutation is estimated to be the cause of adrenal insufficiency in approximately 35% of patients with idiopathic Addison's disease and should be considered in the differential diagnosis of any male with adrenal insufficiency.[3] Most patients develop symptoms of weakness, spasticity, and distal polyneuropathy and may also develop emotional lability, mania, or psychosis.[4] Bladder dysfunction is a common manifestation of adrenomyeloneuropathy and can be a presenting symptom of this disease

Relatives of an Affected Patient

After diagnosis, it is important for the patient's pedigree to be analyzed and those at risk have diagnostic blood work to determine if they have the disease. (The test checks for very long chain fatty acids in the blood, and will also detect most female carriers, but further testing may be required to detect all female carriers). The early identification of affected males is particularly important, as Adrenal hormone replacement therapy is critical and may be life saving. If a family member tests positive, they can receive this treatment, and prevent certain life threatening symptoms, such as an Addisonian crisis.

ADRENAL FATIGUE

Adrenal fatigue or hypoadrenia is a putative health disorder in which the adrenal glands are claimed to be exhausted and unable to produce adequate quantities of hormones, primarily cortisol. The term "adrenal fatigue" is a label sometimes applied to a collection of non-specific medically unexplained symptoms, but it is not a medical condition recognized by mainstream institutions. Adrenal dysfunction as identified by such institutions is termed adrenal insufficiency or Addison's Disease.[1]

The term "adrenal fatigue" is used by some practitioners of alternative medicine, who claim that adrenal fatigue is too mild to be picked up on standard blood tests of adrenal function. The concept has given rise to an industry of dietary supplements claiming to treat this supposed syndrome.

I am 31 years old and recently took an Adrenal Stress Index due to chronic fatigue. My cortisol levels severly depressed. I was diagnosed with adrenal fatigue. I've been prescribed 5 mg Hydrocortisone to take once at 7 am, noon, and 4 pm as well as 5 mg DHEA once daily. I wanted to start out conservatively because I'm afraid of adverse side effects. Has anyone had

any side effects from Hydrocortisone and DHEA? Has anyone been successful in treating Adrenal Fatigue?

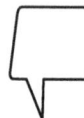

I'm 30, and have had chronic fatigue syndrome for 8 years, and was recently diagnosed with Adrenal Insufficiency, via an insulin tolerance test. Have you tried other adrenal supplements first? Licorice root is what I started on when I had severe adrenal symptoms. It really picked me up in a big way, but its effect wore off and I needed more until I got bad enough to need hydrocortisone (cortef). I haven't been on it long and am on a bit of a rollercoaster, but so far it's provided some benefits such as really helping my constant hypoglycemia, stopped the freezing cold inner shakes I was having, etc. I have periods of feeling a lot better, but so far they're only small windows. The DHEA can and does help a lot of people with adrenal fatigue, adrenal insufficiency, and Addison's.

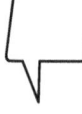

Three 5mg doses of hydrocortisone and 5mg of DHEA is very conservative. It will take the DHEA several weeks to kick in, and the hydrocortisone will take some time as well. Many people don't see an improvement for many months. That dose may be too low to recharge your system and you may *need higher doses to get feeling normal and then cut back a bit.*

AUTOIMMUNE ADRENALITIS

Autoimmune adrenalitis is a form of adrenalitis which is primarily caused by an autoimmune condition.

It is the most common cause of adrenocortical insufficiency in countries where tuberculosis is well controlled.[1]

It can be a component of Autoimmune polyendocrine syndrome type 1 or Autoimmune polyendocrine syndrome type 2, but it can also present as an isolated condition.

The incidence of autoimmune adrenalitis is estimated as one in 20,000.

ADDISON'S DISEASE

CORTISOL

Cortisol is a corticosteroid hormone or glucocorticoid produced by the adrenal cortex, that is part of the adrenal gland (in the zona fasciculata and the zona reticularis of the adrenal cortex). It is usually referred to as the "stress hormone" as it is involved in response to stress and anxiety, controlled by corticotropin releasing hormone. It increases blood pressure and blood sugar, and reduces immune responses. Various synthetic forms of cortisol are used to treat a variety of different illnesses. The most well-known of these are a natural metabolic intermediary of cortisol named hydrocortisone. When first introduced as a treatment for rheumatoid arthritis, hydrocortisone was referred to as Compound E.

I had Cushing's disease 18 years ago and now my cortisol level is low. I seem to have the same symptoms as Addison's disease... is this something I should worry about?

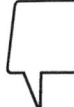

Yes you should definitely get your cortisol level done, and get some steroids for the possible Addison's.

Physiology

The amount of cortisol present in the blood undergoes diurnal variation, with the highest levels present in the early morning, and the lowest levels present around midnight, or 3–5 hours after the onset of sleep. Information about the light/dark cycle is transmitted from the retina to the paired suprachiasmatic nuclei in the hypothalamus. The pattern is not present at birth (estimates of when it starts vary from two weeks to nine months).[1]

Changed patterns of serum cortisol levels have been observed in connection with abnormal adrenocorticotropic hormone levels, clinical depression, psychological stress, and such physiological stressors as hypoglycemia, illness, fever, trauma, surgery, fear, pain, physical exertion or extremes of temperature.

There is also significant individual variation, although a given person tends to have consistent rhythms.

My thyroid test came back good, but why do I still have symptoms? The doctor said all my tests came back in normal range. This all started one month ago with high blood pressure and my blood test then came back with low numbers of my thyroid. I saw an endocrinologist; he said I

have subclinical Hyperthyroidism. I'm frustrated because I still have this annoying pain and am not feeling good.

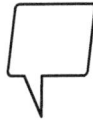

Has the doctor checked your adrenal function? I have found that my thyroid hormones can be ideal and so long as my adrenals are producing the right amount of cortisol, I'm fantastic. The moment I begin to feel like rubbish again, I know it's my adrenals.

A lot of doctors overlook the adrenals and if your cortisol levels are not right, no amount of thyroid medication will make that better. Often adrenal and thyroid issues go hand in hand and their symptoms are very similar.

So I'd say ask your doctor to do an adrenal check. A saliva test is best where they check your cortisol levels throughout the day e.g.: 6am, 12noon, 6pm and 10pm. You get a kit and you do it from home. A morning only test is not good enough as some people produce sufficient cortisol first thing in the morning, but by mid morning their cortisol levels have nose dived and gone down the toilet.

HEALTHSCOUTER

Effects

In normal release, cortisol (like other glucocorticoid agents) has widespread actions which help restore homeostasis after stress. (These normal endogenous functions are the basis for the physiological consequences of chronic stress - prolonged cortisol secretion.). It has been proposed that its primary function is to inversely mobilize the immune system to fight potassium-depleting diarrhea diseases.[2]

Can adrenal glands cause sudden spike of blood pressure and anxiety?

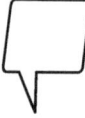
Too high levels of cortisol, which the adrenals produce, can cause high blood pressure and anxiety, but these symptoms can also be caused by a whole host of other things. I imagine if you are taking supplements with sheep adrenal extract and you don't have low cortisol levels, you will have unpleasant effects of high cortisol.

Insulin

Cortisol counteracts insulin by increasing gluconeogenesis and promotes breakdown of lipids (lipolysis), and proteins, and mobilization of extrahepatic amino acids and ketone bodies. This leads to increased circulating glucose concentrations (in the blood) by increasing gluconeogenesis. There is an increased glycogen breakdown in the liver.[3] Prolonged cortisol secretion causes hyperglycemia. The reason why in vivo experiments seem to deny this is that cortisone (a cortisol metabolite) greatly inhibits insulin. So the cortisone-cortisol equilibrium may explain why in vivo experiments contradict the cortisol effect.[4] Cortisol does cause serum glucose to rise, but this is probably an indirect effect caused by stimulation of amino acid degradation, especially that derived from collagen in the skin. In rats, loss of collagen from skin, caused by cortisol, is ten times greater than loss from any other tissue.[5]

Amino acids

Cortisol raises the free amino acids in the serum. It does this by inhibiting collagen formation, decreasing amino acid uptake by muscle, and inhibiting protein synthesis.[6] Cortisol (as opticortinol) probably inversely inhibits IgA precursor cells in the intestines of calves.[7] Cortisol also inhibits IgA in serum, as it does IgM, but not IgE.[8]

Gastric secretion

Cortisol stimulates gastric acid secretion.[9] Gastric acid secretion would increase loss of potassium into the stomach during diarrhea as well as acid loss. Cortisol's only direct effect on the hydrogen ion excretion of the kidneys is to stimulate excretion of ammonium ion by inactivation of renal glutaminase enzyme.[10] Net chloride secretion in the intestines is inversely decreased by cortisol in vitro (methylprednisolone).[11]

Sodium

Cortisol inhibits loss of sodium from small intestines of mammals.[12] However, sodium depletion does not affect cortisol,[13] so cortisol is not used to regulate serum sodium. Cortisol's purpose may originally have been centered around moving sodium because cortisol is used to stimulate sodium inward for fresh water fish and outward for salt-water fish.[14]

Potassium

Sodium load augments the intense potassium excretion by cortisol, and corticosterone is comparable to cortisol in this case.[15] In order for potassium to move out of the cell, cortisol moves in an equal number of sodium ions.[16] It can be seen that this should make pH regulation much easier, unlike the normal potassium deficiency situation in which about 2 sodium ions move in for each three potassium ions that move out, which is closer to the deoxycorticosterone effect. Nevertheless, cortisol consistently causes alkalosis of the serum, while in a deficiency pH does not change. Perhaps this may be for the purpose of bringing serum pH to a value most optimum for some of the immune enzymes during infection in those times when cortisol declines. Potassium is also blocked from loss in the kidneys directly somewhat by decline of cortisol (9 alpha fluorohydrocortisone).[17]

Water

Cortisol also acts as an anti-diuretic hormone. Half the intestinal diuresis is so controlled.[12] Kidney diuresis is also controlled by cortisol in dogs. The decline in water excretion upon decline of cortisol (dexamethasone) in dogs is probably due to inverse stimulation of antidiuretic hormone (ADH or arginine vasopressin), the inverse stimulation of which is not overridden by water loading.[18] Humans also use this mechanism[19] and other different animal mechanisms operate in the same direction.

Copper

It is probable that increasing copper availability for immune purposes is the reason many copper enzymes are stimulated to an extent which is often 50% of their total potential by cortisol.[20] This includes lysyl oxidase, an enzyme which is used to cross link collagen and elastin.[21] Particularly valuable for immunity is the stimulation of superoxide dismutase by cortisol[22] since this copper enzyme is almost certainly used by the body to permit superoxide to poison bacteria. Cortisol causes an inverse four- or fivefold decrease of metallothionein, a copper storage protein, in mice[23] (however rodents do not synthesize cortisol themselves). This may be to furnish more copper for ceruloplasmin synthesis or release of free copper. Cortisol has an opposite effect on alpha aminoisobuteric acid than on the other amino acids.[24] If alpha aminoisobuteric acid is used to transport copper through the cell wall, this anomaly would possibly be explained.

Immune system

Cortisol can weaken the activity of the immune system. Cortisol prevents proliferation of T-cells by rendering the interleukin-2 producer T-cells unresponsive to interleukin-1 (IL-1), and unable to produce the T-cell growth factor.[25] Cortisol has a negative feedback effect on interleukin-1[26] which must be especially useful in combating diseases, such as the endotoxin bacteria, that gain an advantage by forcing the hypothalamus to secrete a hormone called corticotropin releasing hormone. The suppressor cells are not affected by glucosteroid response modifying factor,[27] so that the effective set point for the immune cells may be even higher than the set point for physiological processes. It reflects leukocyte redistribution to lymph nodes, bone marrow, and skin. Acute administration of corticosterone (the endogenous Type I and Type II receptor agonist), or RU28362 (a specific Type II receptor agonist), to adrenalectomized animals induced changes in leukocyte distribution. Natural killer cells are not affected by cortisol.[28]

Bone metabolism

It lowers bone formation thus favoring development of osteoporosis in the long term. Cortisol moves potassium out of cells in exchange for an equal number of sodium ions as mentioned above.[29] This can cause a major problem with the hyperkalemia of metabolic shock from surgery. Cortisol reduces calcium absorption in the intestine.[30]

Memory

It cooperates with epinephrine (adrenaline) to create memories of short-term emotional events;

this is the proposed mechanism for storage of flash bulb memories, and may originate as a means to remember what to avoid in the future. However, long-term exposure to cortisol results in damage to cells in the hippocampus.[31] This damage results in impaired learning. The desirability of inhibiting activity during infection is no doubt the reason why cortisol is responsible for creating euphoria.[32] The desirability of not disturbing tissues weakened by infection or of not cutting off their blood supply could explain the inhibition of pain widely observed for cortisol.

Additional effects

- It increases blood pressure by increasing the sensitivity of the vasculature to epinephrine and norepinephrine. In the absence of cortisol, widespread vasodilation occurs.

- It inhibits the secretion of corticotropin-releasing hormone (CRH), resulting in feedback inhibition of adrenocorticotropic hormone (Adrenocorticotropic hormone or corticotropin) secretion. Some researchers believe that this normal feedback system may become dysregulated when animals are exposed to chronic stress.

- It allows for the kidneys to produce hypotonic urine.

- It has anti-inflammatory effects by reducing histamine secretion and stabilizing lysosomal membranes. The stabilization of lysosomal membranes prevents their rupture, thereby preventing damage to healthy tissues.

- It stimulates hepatic detoxification by inducing tryptophan oxygenase (to reduce serotonin levels in the brain), glutamine synthase (reduce glutamate and ammonia levels in the brain), cytochrome P-450 hemoprotein (mobilizes arachidonic acid), and metallothionein (reduces heavy metals in the body).

- In addition to the effects caused by cortisol binding to the glucocorticoid receptor, because of its molecular similarity to aldosterone, it also binds to the mineralocorticoid receptor. Aldosterone and cortisol have similar affinity for the mineralocorticoid receptor however, glucocorticoids circulate at roughly 100 times the level of mineralocorticoids. An enzyme exists in mineralocorticoid target tissues to prevent overstimulation by glucocorticoids and allow selective mineralocorticoid action. This enzyme, 11-beta hydroxysteroid dehydrogenase type II (Protein:HSD11B2), catalyzes the deactivation of glucocorticoids to 11-dehydro metabolites.

Binding

Most serum cortisol, all but about 4%, is bound to proteins including corticosteroid binding globulin **(CBG),** and serum albumin. Only free cortisol is available to most receptors.

Regulation

The primary control of cortisol is the pituitary gland peptide, adrenocorticotropic hormone (ACTH). Adrenocorticotropic hormone probably controls cortisol by controlling movement of calcium into the cortisol secreting target cells.[33] Adrenocorticotropic hormone is in turn controlled by the hypothalamic peptide, corticotropin releasing hormone (CRH), which is under nervous control. Corticotropin releasing hormone acts synergistically with arginine vasopressin, angiotensin II, and epinephrine.[34] When activated macrophages start to secrete interleukin-1 (IL-1), which synergistically with corticotropin releasing hormone increases adrenocorticotropic hormone,[35] T-cells also secrete glucosteroid response modifying factor (GRMF or GAF) as well as IL-1, both of which increase the amount of cortisol required to inhibit almost all the immune cells.[27] Thus immune cells take over their own regulation, but at a higher cortisol set point. Even so, the rise of cortisol in diarrheic calves is minimal over healthy calves and drops below with time.[36] The cells do not lose all of the fight or flight override because of interleukin-1's synergism with corticotropin releasing hormone. Cortisol even has a negative feedback effect on interleukin-1[37] which must be especially useful against those diseases which gain an advantage by forcing the hypothalamus to secrete too much corticotropin releasing hormone, such as the endotoxin bacteria. The suppressor immune cells are not affected by glucosteroid response modifying factor,[27] so that the effective set point for the immune cells may be even higher than the set point for physiological processes. glucosteroid response modifying factor primarily affects the liver rather than the kidneys for some physiological processes.[38]

A high potassium media, which stimulates aldosterone secretion in vitro, also stimulates cortisol secretion from the fasciculata zone of dog adrenals[39] unlike corticosterone, upon which potassium has no effect.[40] Potassium loading increases adrenocorticotropic hormone and cortisol in people also.[41] This is no doubt the reason why a potassium deficiency causes cortisol to decline (as just mentioned) and why a potassium deficiency causes a decrease in conversion of 11deoxycortisol to cortisol.[42] This probably contributes to the pain in rheumatoid arthritis since cell potassium is always low in that disease.[43]

I am pretty 'new' to Addison's. I have a huge problem with my legs; I have to sit with them up 50% of the time because I get fluid in them. Is that because I get too much medicine?

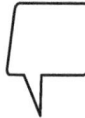
Yes, that could indeed be a sign of too much cortisol. You need to call you physician and see if they can check your levels. I was told a few years ago that you can develop Graves if you have too much cortisol.

Factors affecting cortisol levels

Factors generally reducing cortisol levels

- Magnesium supplementation decreases serum cortisol levels after aerobic exercise,[44][45] but not in resistance training.[46]

- Omega 3 fatty acids, in a dose dependent manner,[47] can lower cortisol release influenced by mental stress[48] by suppressing the synthesis of interleukin-1 and 6 and enhance the synthesis of interleukin-2, where the former promote higher corticotropin releasing hormone release. Omega 6 fatty acids, on the other hand, acts inversely on interleukin synthesis.

- Music therapy can reduce cortisol levels in certain situations.[49]

- Massage therapy can reduce cortisol.[50]

- Laughing and the experience of humor can lower cortisol levels.[51]

- Makeup reduces cortisol levels in a mental stress situation.[52]

- Soy derived Phosphatidylserine interacts with cortisol but the right dosage is still unclear.[53][54]

- Vitamin C may slightly blunt cortisol release in response to a mental stressor.[55]

I had a visit with an endocrinologist last month and will visit with him again at the end of the month. I originally wanted to see him because I thought I might have Hashimoto's Thyroiditis. I've had Fibromyalgia for years and diagnosed with some kind of systematic rheumatic condition that almost fit the criteria for Lupus about two years ago and thought I might be having thyroid issues because of some recent lab work. I have antibodies that indicate possible Hashimoto's,

but an adrenal nodule was found on a CT scan a couple of years ago that I also discussed with the endocrinologist. Needless to say, he's run a bunch of blood work, a 24 urine, and an MRI of my adrenal glands.

So far, I think the lab work is indicating that my aldosterone is low. I think it was supposed to be in the 20's and came in at 5. I had the ACTH test done at 2:00 in the afternoon. The start was 19 and then jumped to 45.6 in an hour. I have no idea if that is normal. I have received the 24 hour urine results back yet. He was testing metanephrines and catecholamines. The MRI indicated a possible adenoma.

What concerns me is my increased fatigue and the darkening of the skin of my toes, knuckles, elbows, and scars. Also - because of the lupus, I try to avoid the sun as much as possible but still seem to be darker than normal. I sometimes feel a bit dizzy and have been trying to make sure that I don't wait too long to eat between meals. I'm also the only one I know of in my family that does not have high blood pressure. Occasionally my heart rate is high. I almost always have some form of abdominal pain that I attributed to irritable bowel syndrome. I also crave salt and *just feel blah. When I was younger I had so much more energy. Now at 35 I spend a majority of my time resting when not working or rushing around to do other things. Any input would be greatly appreciated.*

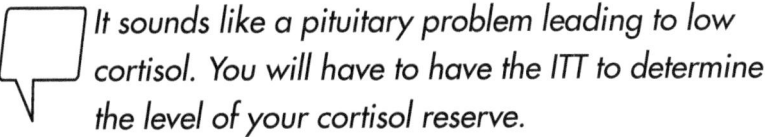It sounds like a pituitary problem leading to low cortisol. You will have to have the ITT to determine the level of your cortisol reserve.

Factors generally increasing cortisol levels

- Caffeine may increase cortisol levels.[56]

- Sleep deprivation increases cortisol levels.[57]

- Intense (high VO2 max) or prolonged physical exercise stimulate cortisol release in order to increase gluconeogenesis and maintain blood glucose.[58] Proper nutrition[59] and high-level conditioning[60] can help stabilize cortisol release.

- Val/Val variation of the BDNF gene in men, and the Val/Met variation in women is associated with increased salivary cortisol in a stressful situation.[61]

- Hypoestrogenism and melatonin supplementation increases cortisol levels in postmenopausal women.[62]

- Burnout is associated with higher cortisol levels.[63]

- Subcutaneous adipose tissue regenerates cortisol from cortisone.[64]

- Anorexia nervosa increases cortisol levels.[65]

- Black tea may speed up recovery from a high cortisol condition.[66][67]

- The serotonin receptor gene 5HTR2C is associated with increased cortisol production in men.[68]

- Oral contraceptives increase cortisol levels in young women who perform whole-body resistance exercise training.[69]

- Commuting increases cortisol levels, related to the length of the trip, the amount of effort involved and the predictability of the trip.[70]

Pharmacology

Hydrocortisone is the pharmaceutical term for cortisol used for oral administration, intravenous injection, or topical application. It is used as an immunosuppressive drug, given by injection in the treatment of severe allergic reactions such as anaphylaxis and angioedema, in place of prednisolone in patients who need steroid treatment but cannot take oral medication, and peri-operatively in patients on long-term steroid treatment to prevent an Addisonian crisis. It may be used topically for allergic rashes, eczema, psoriasis and certain other inflammatory skin conditions. It may also be injected into inflamed joints resulting from diseases such as gout.

Compared to prednisolone, hydrocortisone is about 1/4 the strength for the anti-inflammatory effect, while Dexamethasone is about 40 times as strong as hydrocortisone. For side effects, see corticosteroid and prednisolone.

Hydrocortisone creams and ointments are available without prescription in strengths ranging from 0.05% to 2.5%, depending on local regulations, with stronger forms available with prescriptions only. Covering the skin after application increases the absorption and effect. Such enhancement is sometimes prescribed, but otherwise should be avoided to prevent over-dosing and systemic impacts.

Advertising for the dietary supplement CortiSlim originally (and falsely) claimed that it contributed to weight loss by blocking cortisol. The manufacturer was fined $1.2 million by the Federal Trade Commission in 2007 for false advertising, and no longer claims in their marketing that CortiSlim is a cortisol antagonist.[71]

HEALTHSCOUTER

I'm a 33-year-old male with Hashimoto's Thyroiditis. I've had several blood tests for ACTH, Cortisol and a number of other things. My early morning ACTH is almost always elevated while my cortisol is always normal to high-normal (both checked in the same draws). In the evening, both my ACTH and cortisol drop down to normal range.

The ratio of adrenocorticotropic hormone versus cortisol goes to NORMAL in the afternoon, but is way out of whack in the morning. My body wants more cortisol in the morning but has a difficult time producing it at that time.

I think I have adrenal fatigue (although doctors don't believe in this), but not quite yet Addison's disease. I think it will lead to this eventually if it goes unsolved.

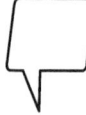
I agree you seem to have adrenal fatigue and a saliva cortisol test would probably confirm it. It's also probably why you couldn't tolerate the natural thyroid hormones. It sounds like you might need some hydrocortisone to get the adrenals a rest and allow them to heal.

ADDISON'S DISEASE

Biochemistry

Biosynthesis

Cortisol is synthesized from cholesterol. The synthesis takes place in the *zona fasciculata* of the cortex of the adrenal glands. (The name *cortisol* comes from *cortex*.) While the adrenal cortex also produces aldosterone (in the *zona glomerulosa*) and some sex hormones (in the *zona reticularis*), cortisol is its main secretion. The medulla of the adrenal gland lies under the cortex and mainly secretes the catecholamines, adrenaline (epinephrine) and noradrenaline (norepinephrine) under sympathetic stimulation (more epinephrine is produced than norepinephrine, in a ratio 4:1).

The synthesis of cortisol in the adrenal gland is stimulated by the anterior lobe of the pituitary gland with adrenocorticotropic hormone (ACTH); production of adrenocorticotropic hormone is in turn stimulated by corticotropin-releasing hormone (CRH), released by the hypothalamus. adrenocorticotropic hormone increases the concentration of cholesterol in the inner mitochondrial membrane (via regulation of STAR (steroidogenic acute regulatory) protein). adrenocorticotropic hormone also stimulates the main rate-limiting step in cortisol synthesis where cholesterol is converted to pregnenolone, catalyzed by Cytochrome P450SCC (side chain cleavage enzyme).[72]

Metabolism

Cortisol is metabolized by the 11-beta hydroxysteroid dehydrogenase system (11-beta HSD), which consists of two enzymes: 11-beta HSD1 and 11-beta HSD2.

- *11-beta HSD1* utilizes the cofactor NADPH to convert biologically inert cortisone to biologically active cortisol.

- *11-beta HSD2* utilizes the cofactor NAD+ to convert cortisol to cortisone.

Overall the net effect is that 11-beta HSD1 serves to increase the local concentrations of biologically active cortisol in a given tissue, while 11-beta HSD2 serves to decrease the local concentrations of biologically active cortisol.

Cortisol is also metabolized into 5-alpha tetrahydrocortisol (5-alpha THF) and 5-beta tetrahydrocortisol (5-beta THF), reactions for which 5-alpha reductase and 5-beta reductase are the rate-limiting factors, respectively. 5-beta reductase is also the rate-limiting factor in the conversion of cortisone to tetrahydrocortisone (THE).

The CA3 area of hippocampus (memory) is affected by cortisol.

An alteration in 11-beta HSD1 has been suggested to play a role in the pathogenesis of obesity, hypertension, and insulin resistance, sometimes referred to the metabolic syndrome.

An alteration in 11-beta HSD2 has been implicated in essential hypertension and is known to lead to the syndrome of apparent mineralocorticoid excess (SAME).

REFERENCES – ADDISON'S DISEASE

1. Addison disease at Dorland's Medical Dictionary

2. Thomas Addison (1855) (HTML reprint). *On The Constitutional And Local Effects Of Disease Of The Supra-Renal Capsules.* London: Samuel Highley. http://www.wehner.org/addison/x1.htm.

3. Ten S, New M, Maclaren N (2001). "Clinical review 130: Addison's disease 2001". *J. Clin. Endocrinol. Metab.* **86** (7): 2909–22. doi:10.1210/jc.86.7.2909. PMID 11443143. http://jcem.endojournals.org/cgi/content/full/86/7/2909.

4. Patnaik MM, Deshpande AK (May 2008). "Diagnosis--Addison's disease secondary to tuberculosis of the adrenal glands". *Clin Med Res* **6** (1): 29. doi:10.3121/cmr.2007.754a. PMID 18591375. PMC: 2442022. http://www.clinmedres.org/cgi/pmidlookup?view=long&pmid=18591375.

5. James, William; Berger, Timothy; Elston, Dirk (2005). *Andrews' Diseases of the Skin: Clinical Dermatology.* (10th ed.). Saunders. ISBN 0721629210.

6. Addison's Disease National Endocrine and Metabolic Diseases Information Service. Retrieved on 26 October 2007.

7. Lauretti, S; Casucci, G; Santeisanio, F (1996), "X-linked adrenoleukodystrophy is a frequent cause of idiopathic Addison's disease in young adult male patient.", *J Clin Endocrinol Metab* **81**: 470–474.

8. Wang L, Yang J (2008). "Tuberculous Addison's disease mimics malignancy in FDG-PET images" ([dead link]). *Intern. Med.* **47** (19): 1755–6. doi:10.2169/internalmedicine.47.1348. PMID 18827432. http://joi.jlc.jst.go.jp/JST.JSTAGE/internalmedicine/47.1348?from=PubMed.

9. "Addison Disease • Health information regarding this hormonal (endocrine) disorder on MedicineNet.com". http://www.medicinenet.com/addison_disease/article.htm. Retrieved on 2007-07-25.

10. "eMedicine - Addison Disease : Article by Sylvester Odeke". http://www.emedicine.com/med/topic42.htm. Retrieved on 2007-07-25.

11. "medhelp". http://www.medhelp.org/www/nadf3.htm. Retrieved on 2007-07-25.

12. Volpé, Robert (1990). *Autoimmune Diseases of the Endocrine System.* CRC Press. pp. 299. ISBN 0849368499.

13. "Dog Days Of Science". http://grants.nih.gov/grants/policy/air/dog_days.htm. Retrieved on 2008-09-01.

14. Nicholas JA, Burstein CL, Umberger CJ, Wilson PD (November 1955). "Management of adrenocortical insufficiency during surgery". *AMA Arch Surg* **71** (5): 737–42. PMID 13268224.

15. Owen, David (May 2003). "Diseased, demented, depressed: serious illness in Heads of State". *QJM: an International Journal of Medicine* (Oxford University Press) **96** (5): 325–36. doi:10.1093/qjmed/hcg061. PMID 12702781. http://qjmed.oxfordjournals.org/cgi/content/full/96/5/325.

16. Dallek, Robert (2003). *An Unfinished Life: John F. Kennedy, 1917-1963*. London: Penguin Books. pp. 105, 731. ISBN 978-0141015354.

17. "The Australian Addison's Disease Association". http://www.addisons.org.au/core.htm?page=/awareness/awarenessweek.htm. Retrieved on 2007-07-25.

18. Marsden, Brian (1997-07-18). "Eugene Shoemaker (1928–1997)" (HTML). *Comet Shoemaker-Levy Collision with Jupiter*. Jet Propulsion Laboratory. http://www2.jpl.nasa.gov/sl9/news81.html. Retrieved on 2007-07-25.

19. Jones, Terry. "Patron Saints Index: Blessed Elizabeth of the Trinity". http://saints.sqpn.com/sainte46.htm. Retrieved on 2008-05-04.

20. Upfal, Annette (2005). "Jane Austen's lifelong health problems and final illness: New evidence points to a fatal Hodgkin's disease and excludes the widely accepted Addison's". *Medical Humanities* (BMJ Publishing Group Ltd) **31**: 3–11. doi:10.1136/jmh.2004.000193. http://mh.bmj.com/cgi/content/full/31/1/3.

21. L. Williams et al. (1991). "The Nineteenth Century: Victorian Period". *The Year's Work in English Studies* (Oxford University Press) **72** (1): pp. 314–360. doi:10.1093/ywes/72.1.314. http://ywes.oxfordjournals.org/cgi/content/long/72/1/314.

22. Wright, Lawrence (2006). *The Looming Tower*. New York City: Alfred A. Knopf, Inc. p. 139. ISBN 978-0375414862.

REFERENCES – ADRENAL INSUFFICIENCY

1. Eileen K. Corrigan (2007). "Adrenal Insufficiency (Secondary Addison's or Addison's Disease)". *NIH Publication No. 90-3054.* http://www.pituitary.org/disorders/addisons_disease.aspx.

2. MeSH *Adrenal+Insufficiency*

3. Ten S, New M, Maclaren N (2001). "Clinical review 130: Addison's disease 2001". *J. Clin. Endocrinol. Metab.* **86** (7): 2909–22. doi:10.1210/jc.86.7.2909. PMID 12899587. http://jcem.endojournals.org/cgi/content/full/86/7/2909.

4. Ashley B. Grossman, MD (2007). "Addison's Disease". *Adrenal Gland Disorders.* http://www.merck.com/mmhe/sec13/ch164/ch164b.html.

5. Brender E, Lynm C, Glass RM (2005). "JAMA patient page. Adrenal insufficiency". *JAMA* **294** (19): 2528. doi:10.1001/jama.294.19.2528. PMID 16287965. http://jama.ama-assn.org/cgi/content/full/294/19/2528.

6. "Dorlands Medical Dictionary:adrenal insufficiency". http://www.mercksource.com/pp/us/cns/cns_hl_dorlands_split.jsp?pg=/ppdocs/us/common/dorlands/dorland/four/000053970.htm.

7. "Secondary Adrenal Insufficiency: Adrenal Disorders: Merck Manual Professional". http://www.merck.com/mmpe/sec12/ch153/ch153c.html.

8. "hypopituitary". 2006. http://www.webmd.com/a-to-z-guides/hypopituitary.

9. Thomas A Wilson, MD (2007). "Adrenal Insufficiency". *Adrenal Gland Disorders.* http://www.emedicine.com/PED/topic47.htm.

10. Thomas A Wilson, MD (1999). *Adrenoleukodystrophy.* http://healthlink.mcw.edu/article/921176192.html.

ADDISON'S DISEASE

REFERENCES – ADRENOCORTICOTROPIC HORMONE STIMULATION TEST

1. Dorin RI, Qualls CR, Crapo LM (2003). "Diagnosis of adrenal insufficiency" (PDF). *Ann. Intern. Med.* **139** (3): 194–204. PMID 12899587. http://www.annals.org/cgi/reprint/139/3/194.pdf.

2. Elizabeth H. Holt, MD, PhD (2008). *adrenocorticotropic hormone (cosyntropin) stimulation test.* http://www.nlm.nih.gov/medlineplus/ency/article/003696.htm.

3. unknown. "adrenocorticotropic hormone Stimulation Test" (PDF). APPENDIX – *Endocrinology.* http://www.wardelab.com/Appendix09_adrenocorticotropic hormonea.pdf.

4. unknown (PDF). *Synacthen Test.* http://www.stgeorges.nhs.uk/docs/leaflets/synacthen.pdf.

5. unknown. GENERIC NAME: COSYNTROPIN - INJECTABLE *(koe-sin-TROW-pin).* http://www.medicinenet.com/cosyntropin-injectable/article.htm.

6. unknown (2006). *adrenocorticotropic hormone (Cortrosyn) stimulation test.* http://adam.about.com/encyclopedia/adrenocorticotropic hormone-Cortrosyn-stimulation-test.htm.

7. Evangelia Charmandari, M.D., and George P. Chrousos, M.D.. *ADRENAL INSUFFICIENCY Chapter 13.* http://www.endotext.org/adrenal/adrenal13/adrenalframe13.htm.

8. Abdu TA; Elhadd TA; Neary R; Clayton RN (1999). "Comparison of the low dose short synacthen test (1 microg), the conventional dose short synacthen test (250 microg), and the insulin tolerance test for assessment of the hypothalamic-pituitary-adrenal axis in patients with pituitary disease.". *The Journal of clinical endocrinology and metabolism* **84**: 838. doi:10.1210/jc.84.3.838. http://www.medscape.com/medline/abstract/10084558?src=emed_ckb_ref_0.

9. K. Pagana, PhD, RN and T. Pagana, MD, FACS. Mosby's Diagnostic and Laboratory Test Reference 2nd ed: Adrenocorticotropic hormone stimulation test. pp. 17.

10. K. Pagana, PhD, RN and T. Pagana, MD, FACS. *Mosby's Diagnostic and Lab Test Reference 2nd ed: Aldosterone, Cortisol.* pp. 29 and 260.

11. unknown (2006). *Aldosterone in Blood.* http://www.webmd.com/a-to-z-guides/aldosterone.

12. Emily D. Szmuilowicz, Gail K. Adler, Jonathan S. Williams, Dina E.Green, Tham M. Yao, Paul N. Hopkins and Ellen W. Seely (2006). "Relationship between Aldosterone and Progesterone in the Human Menstrual Cycle". *Journal of Clinical Endocrinology & Metabolism* **91** (10): 3981–3987. doi:10.1210/jc.2006-1154. http://jcem.endojournals.org/cgi/content/full/91/10/3981.

13. unknown. *adrenocorticotropic hormone Rapid Stimulation Test (Cortrosyn, Cosyntropin).* http://www.clinlabnavigator.com/Tests/adrenocorticotropic hormoneRapidStimulationTest.html.
14. NIDDK's Office of Health Research Reports. *Addison's disease.* http://endocrine.niddk.nih.gov/pubs/addison/addison.htm.
15. Ashley B. Grossman, MD (2007). "Addison's Disease". *Endocrine and Metabolic Disorders.* http://www.merck.com/mmpe/print/sec12/ch153/ch153b.html.
16. Lynnette K Nieman, MD (2008). *Corticotropin-releasing hormone stimulation test.* http://www.uptodate.com/patients/content/topic.do?topicKey=~L8psmoE71_MEP.
17. unknown. *Role of adrenocorticotropic hormone in Regulation and Action of Adrenocorticoids.* pp. 7 of 52. http://www.lib.mcg.edu/edu/eshuphysio/program/section5/5ch7/s5ch7_7.htm.
18. unknown. *Aldosterone and Renin.* http://www.labtestsonline.org/understanding/analytes/aldosterone/test.html.
19. L.A. Cunningham and M.A. Holzwarth (1988). "Vasoactive intestinal peptide stimulates adrenal aldosterone and corticosterone secretion". *Endocrinology* **122:** 2090–2097. PMID 3359977. http://endo.endojournals.org/cgi/content/abstract/122/5/2090.
20. Jardena J. Puder, Pamela U. Freda, Robin S. Goland, Michel Ferin,and Sharon L. Wardlaw. "[http://jcem.endojournals.org/cgi/reprint/85/6/2184.pdf Stimulatory Effects of Stress on Gonadotropin Secretion in Estrogen-Treated Women*]" (PDF). *The Journal of Clinical Endocrinology & Metabolism* **85:** 2184–2188. http://jcem.endojournals.org/cgi/reprint/85/6/2184.pdf.
21. unknown. *adrenocorticotropic hormone Stimulation Test for 21-Hydroxylase*

REFERENCES – ADRENOLEUKYDYSTROPHY

1. James, William D.; Berger, Timothy G.; et al. (2006). *Andrews' Diseases of the Skin: clinical Dermatology*. Saunders Elsevier. ISBN 0-7216-2921-0.

2. Siemerling E, Creutzfeldt HG (1923). "Bronzekrankheit und sklerosierende Encephalomyelitis". *Arch. Psychiat. Neurokrankh.* **68:** 217–44. doi:10.1007/BF01835678.

3. O'Brien TJ, Gates PG, Byrne E (April 1996). "Symptomatic female heterozygotes for adrenoleukodystrophy: A report of two unrelated cases and review of the literature". *Journal of Clinical Neuroscience : Official Journal of the Neurosurgical Society of Australasia* **3** (2): 166–70. PMID 18638861. http://linkinghub.elsevier.com/retrieve/pii/S0967-5868(96)90012-0.

4. Moser HW, Moser AB, Frayer KK, et al (October 1981). "Adrenoleukodystrophy: increased plasma content of saturated very long chain fatty acids". *Neurology* **31** (10): 1241–9. PMID 7202134.

5. Moser HW, Raymond GV, Dubey P (Dec 2005). "Adrenoleukodystrophy: new approaches to a neurodegenerative disease". *JAMA* **294** (24): 3131–4. doi:10.1001/jama.294.24.3131. PMID 16380594.

6. Bezman L, Moser AB, Raymond GV, Rinaldo P, Watkins PA, Smith KD, Kass NE, Moser HW (April 2001). "Adrenoleukodystrophy: incidence, new mutation rate, and results of extended family screening". *Annals of Neurology* **49** (4): 512–7.

7. Moser HW, Moser AB, Frayer KK, et al (Oct 1981). "Adrenoleukodystrophy: increased plasma content of saturated very long chain fatty acids". *Neurology* **31** (10): 1241–9. PMID 7202134.

8. Mosser J, Douar AM, Sarde CO, et al (Feb 1993). "Putative X-linked adrenoleukodystrophy gene shares unexpected homology with ABC transporters". *Nature* **361** (6414): 726–30. doi:10.1038/361726a0. PMID 8441467.

9. Bezman L, Moser HW (April 1998). "<415::AID-AJMG9>3.0.CO;2-L Incidence of X-linked adrenoleukodystrophy and the relative frequency of its phenotypes". *American Journal of Medical Genetics* **76** (5): 415–9. PMID 9556301. http://dx.doi.org/10.1002/(SICI)1096-8628(19980413)76:5<415::AID-AJMG9>3.0.CO;2-L.

10. Online 'Mendelian Inheritance in Man' (OMIM) ADRENOLEUKODYSTROPHY, AUTOSOMAL NEONATAL FORM -202370

11. Moser, HW; Raymond GV, Lu S-E, Muenz LR, Moser AB, Xu J, Jones RO, Loes DJ, Melhem ER, Dubey P, Bezman L, Brereton NH, Odone A (2005-07). "Follow-up of 89 asymptomatic patients with adrenoleukodystrophy treated with Lorenzo's Oil.". *Archives of Neurology* **62** (7): p. 1073–80. doi:10.1001/archneur.62.7.1073. PMID 16009761.

12. Moser HW, Moser AB, Hollandsworth K, Brereton NH, Raymond GV (Sep 2007). ""Lorenzo's oil" therapy for X-linked adrenoleukodystrophy: rationale and current assessment of efficacy". *J. Mol. Neurosci.* **33** (1): 105–13. doi:10.1007/s12031-007-0041-4. PMID 17901554.
13. Online 'Mendelian Inheritance in Man' (OMIM) Adrenoleukodystrophy - 300100
14. Peters C, Charnas LR, Tan Y, Ziegler RS, Shapiro EG, DeFor T, Grewal SS, Orchard PJ, Abel SL, Goldman AI, Ramsay NK, Dusenbery KE, Loes DJ, Lockman LA, Kato S, Aubourg PR, Moser HW, Krivit W (2004). "Cerebral X-linked adrenoleukodystrophy: the international hematopoietic cell transplantation experience from 1982 to 1999". *Blood* **104** (3): 881-8. PMID 15073029.
15. Beam D, Poe MD, Provenzale JM, Szabolcs P, Martin PL, Prasad V, Parikh S, Driscoll T, Mukundan S, Kurtzberg J, Escolar ML (2007). "Outcomes of unrelated umbilical cord blood transplantation for X-linked adrenoleukodystrophy". *Biol Blood Marrow Transplant* **13** (6): 665-74. PMID 17531776.
16. Yamada T, Shinnoh N, Taniwaki T, et al (September 2000). "Lovastatin does not correct the accumulation of very long-chain fatty acids in tissues of adrenoleukodystrophy protein-deficient mice". *J. Inherit. Metab. Dis.* **23** (6): 607–14. doi:10.1023/A:1005634130286. PMID 11032335. http://www.kluweronline.com/art.pdf?issn=0141-8955&volume=23&page=607.
17. Pai GS, Khan M, Barbosa E, Key LL, Craver JR, Curé JK, Betros R, Singh I (April 2000). "Lovastatin therapy for X-linked adrenoleukodystrophy: clinical and biochemical observations on 12 patients". *Molecular Genetics and Metabolism* **69** (4): 312–22. PMID 10870849. http://linkinghub.elsevier.com/retrieve/pii/S1096719200929779.
18. Tolar J, Orchard PJ, Bjoraker KJ, Ziegler RS, Shapiro EG, Charnas L (Feb 2007). "N-acetyl-L-cysteine improves outcome of advanced cerebral adrenoleukodystrophy". *Bone Marrow Transplant* **39** (4): 211–5. doi:10.1038/sj.bmt.1705571. PMID 17290278.
19. Rizzo WB, Watkins PA, Phillips MW, Cranin D, Campbell B, Avigan J (March 1986). "Adrenoleukodystrophy: oleic acid lowers fibroblast saturated C22-26 fatty acids". *Neurology* **36** (3): 357–61. PMID 3951702. http://www.ncbi.nlm.nih.gov/pubmed/3951702. Retrieved on 7 October 2008.
20. clinicaltrials.gov/
21. "A Phase III Trial of Lorenzo's Oil in Adrenomyeloneuropathy". http://www.clinicaltrials.gov/show/NCT00545597. Retrieved on 2009-06-06.
22. ClinicalTrials.gov NCT00004450
23. "Study of Glyceryl Trierucate and glyceryl trioleate (Lorenzo's Oil) therapy in male children with adrenoleukodystrophy". http://www.clinicaltrials.gov/show/NCT00004418. Retrieved on 2009-06-06.

24. "HSCT for High Risk Inherited Inborn Errors". http://www.clinicaltrials.gov/show/NCT00383448. Retrieved on 2009-06-06.
25. "Boy whose parents made Lorenzo's oil dies at 30". *SFGate.com*. http://www.sfgate.com/cgi-bin/article.cgi?f=/n/a/2008/05/30/national/a165519D26.DTL&tsp=1. Retrieved on 2008-05-30.
26. "About Lorenzo, his Parents, and Oumouri". *The Myelin Project*. http://www.myelin.org/aboutlorenzo.htm. Retrieved on 2006-06-03.

ADDISON'S DISEASE

REFERENCES – ADRENOMYELONEUROPATHY

1. Moser, HW. (1997), "Adrenoleukodystrophy, phenotypes, genetics, pathogenesis and therapy", *Brain* (120): 1485-1508

2. Oelkers, W. (Oct 17), "Current Concepts: Adrenal Insufficiency", *N Engl. J Med* (335): 1206–1212

3. Lauretti, S; Casucci, G; Santeisanio, F (1996), "X-linked adrenoleukodystrophy is a frequent cause of idiopathic Addison's disease in young adult male patient.", *J Clin Endocrinol Metab* **81:** 470–474

4. Rosebush, PI; Garside, S; Levinson, AJ; Mazurek, MF (1999), "The Neuropsychiatry of Adult-Onset Adrenoleukodystrophy", *J Neuropsychiatry Clin Neurosci* (11): 315–327

5. Nanci, Gabriella N.; Collier, Millard J.; Rose, Sheldon H. (2009), "Twenty Years of Dysuria in a Patient with Addison's Disease", *Cases Journal* **2** (7995)

ADDISON'S DISEASE

REFERENCES – ADRENAL FATIGUE

1. "Adrenal fatigue: What causes it?". MayoClinic.com. Mayo Foundation for Medical Education and Research. http://www.mayoclinic.com/health/adrenal-fatigue/AN01583. Retrieved on 2008-08-03.

ADDISON'S DISEASE

REFERENCES – AUTOIMMUNE ADRENALITIS

1. Cotran, Ramzi S.; Kumar, Vinay; Fausto, Nelson; Nelso Fausto; Robbins, Stanley L.; Abbas, Abul K. (2005). *Robbins and Cotran pathologic basis of disease*. St. Louis, Mo: Elsevier Saunders. pp. 1215-6. ISBN 0-7216-0187-1.

2. Eugster, Erica A.; Pescovitz, Ora Hirsch (2004). *Pediatric endocrinology: mechanisms, manifestations and management*. Hagerstwon, MD: Lippincott Williams & Wilkins. pp. 576. ISBN 0-7817-4059-2.

ADDISON'S DISEASE

REFERENCES – CORTISOL

1. de Weerth C, Zijl R, Buitelaar J (2003). "Development of cortisol circadian rhythm in infancy". *Early Hum Dev* **73** (1-2): 39–52. doi:10.1016/S0378-3782(03)00074-4. PMID 12932892.

2. Weber CE (1998) "Cortisol's purpose." Medical Hypotheses 51; 289-292.

3. Freeman, Scott (2002). *Biological Science*. Prentice Hall; 2nd Pkg edition (December 30, 2004). ISBN 0-13-218746-9.

4. Curry DL, Bennett LL (September 1973). "Dynamics of insulin release by perfused rat pancreases: effects of hypophysectomy, growth hormone, adrenocorticotropic hormone, and hydrocortisone". *Endocrinology* **93** (3): 602–9. PMID 4352804.

5. Houck JC, Sharma VK, Patel YM, Gladner JA (October 1968). "Induction of collagenolytic and proteolytic activities by anti-inflammatory drugs in the skin and fibroblast". *Biochem. Pharmacol.* **17** (10): 2081–90. PMID 4301453.

6. Manchester, K.L., "Sites of Hormonal Regulation of Protein Metabolism. p. 229", Mammalian Protein[Munro, H.N., Ed.]. Academic Press, New York. On p273.

7. Husband AJ, Brandon MR, Lascelles AK (October 1973). "The effect of corticosteroid on absorption and endogenous production of immunoglobulins in calves". *Aust J Exp Biol Med Sci* **51** (5): 707–10. PMID 4207041.

8. Posey WC, Nelson HS, Branch B, Pearlman DS (December 1978). "The effects of acute corticosteroid therapy for asthma on serum immunoglobulin levels". *J. Allergy Clin. Immunol.* **62** (6): 340–8. PMID 712020.

9. Soffer, L.J.; Dorfman, R.I.; Gabrilove, J.L,. "The Human Adrenal Gland". Febiger, Phil.

10. Kokshchuk, G.I.; Pakhmurnyi, B.A. (1979) "Role of Glucocorticoids in Regulation of the Acid-Excreting Function of the Kidneys". Fiziol. Z H SSR I.M.I.M. Sechenova 65: 751,.

11. Tai YH, Decker RA, Marnane WG, Charney AN, Donowitz M (May 1981). "Effects of methylprednisolone on electrolyte transport by in vitro rat ileum". *Am. J. Physiol.* **240** (5): G365–70. PMID 6112881.

12. Sandle GI, Keir MJ, Record CO (1981). "The effect of hydrocortisone on the transport of water, sodium, and glucose in the jejunum. Perfusion studies in normal subjects and patients with coeliac disease". *Scand. J. Gastroenterol.* **16** (5): 667–71. PMID 7323700.

13. Mason PA, Fraser R, Morton JJ, Semple PF, Wilson A (August 1977). "The effect of sodium deprivation and of angiotensin II infusion on the peripheral plasma concentrations of 18-hydroxycorticosterone, aldosterone and other corticosteroids in man". *J. Steroid Biochem.* **8** (8): 799–804. PMID 592808.

14. Gorbman, A.; Dickhoff, W.W.; Vigna, S.R.; Clark, N.B.; Muller, A.F,. "Comparative Endocrinology". John Wiley and Sons, New York.

15. Muller AF Oconnor CM, ed. (1958) "An International Symposium on Aldosterone", page 58. Little Brown & Co.

16. KNIGHT RP, KORNFELD DS, GLASER GH, BONDY PK (February 1955). "Effects of intravenous hydrocortisone on electrolytes of serum and urine in man". *J. Clin. Endocrinol. Metab.* **15** (2): 176–81. PMID 13233328.

17. BARGER AC, BERLIN RD, TULENKO JF (June 1958). "Infusion of aldosterone, 9-alpha-fluorohydrocortisone and antidiuretic hormone into the renal artery of normal and adrenalectomized, unanesthetized dogs: effect on electrolyte and water excretion". *Endocrinology* **62** (6): 804–15. PMID 13548099.

18. Boykin J, DeTorrenté A, Erickson A, Robertson G, Schrier RW (October 1978). "Role of plasma vasopressin in impaired water excretion of glucocorticoid deficiency". *J. Clin. Invest.* **62** (4): 738–44. doi:10.1172/JCI109184. PMID 701472.

19. Dingman, J.F.; Gonzalez-Auvert Ahmed, A.B.J.; Akinura, A. (1965) "Antidiuretic Hormone in Adrenal Insufficiency". Journal of Clinical Investigation 44: 1041,.

20. Weber, C.E (1984). "Copper Response to Rheumatoid Arthritis". Medical Hypotheses 15: 333-348, on p337,.

21. Weber, C.E. (1984) "Copper Response to Rheumatoid Arthritis". Medical Hypotheses 15: 333,.on p334.

22. Flohe, L.; Beckman, R.; Giertz, H.; Loschen, G. "Oxygen Centered Free Radicals as Mediators of Inflammation. p. 405", Oxidative Stress (Sies H, ed) Academic Press, New York.

23. Piletz JE, Herschman HR (June 1983). "Hepatic metallothionein synthesis in neonatal Mottled-Brindled mutant mice". *Biochem. Genet.* **21** (5-6): 465–75. PMID 6870774.

24. Chambers, J.W.; Georg, R.H. and Bass, A.D. (1965) "Effect of Hydrocortisone and Insulin on Uptake of Alpha Aminoisobutyric Acid by Isolated Perfused Rat Liver". Mol. Pharmacol. 1: 66,.

25. Palacios R., Sugawara I. (1982). "Hydrocortisone abrogates proliferation of T cells in autologous mixed lymphocyte reaction by rendering the interleukin-2 Producer T cells unresponsive to interleukin-1 and unable to synthesize the T-cell growth factor". *Scand J Immunol* **15** (1): 25–31. doi:10.1111/j.1365-3083.1982.tb00618.x. PMID 6461917.

26. Besedovsky, H.O.; Del Rey, A.; Sorkin, E. (1984) "Integration of Activated Immune Cell Products in Immune Endocrine Feedback Circuits." p. 200 in Leukocytes and Host Defense Vol. 5[Oppenheim, J.J.; Jacobs, D.M., eds]. Alan R. Liss, New York,.

27. Fairchild SS, Shannon K, Kwan E, Mishell RI (February 1984). "T cell-derived glucosteroid response-modifying factor (GRMFT): a unique lymphokine made by normal T lymphocytes and a T cell hybridoma". *J. Immunol.* **132** (2): 821–7. PMID 6228602.

28. Onsrud M, Thorsby E (1981). "Influence of in vivo hydrocortisone on some human blood lymphocyte subpopulations. I. Effect on natural killer cell activity". *Scand. J. Immunol.* **13** (6): 573–9. PMID 7313552.

29. Knight, R.P., Jr. Kornfield, D.S. Glaser, G.H. Bondy, P.K. (1955). "Effects of intravenous hydrocortisone on electrolytes of serum and urine in man". *J Clin Endocrinol Metab* **15** (2): 176–81. PMID 13233328.

30. Shultz TD, Bollman S, Kumar R (June 1982). "Decreased intestinal calcium absorption in vivo and normal brush border membrane vesicle calcium uptake in cortisol-treated chickens: evidence for dissociation of calcium absorption from brush border vesicle uptake". *Proc. Natl. Acad. Sci. U.S.A.* **79** (11): 3542–6. PMID 6954501.

31. Mc Auley MM, Kenny RA, Kirkwood TT, Wilkinson DD, Jones JJ, Miller VM (March 2009). "A Mathematical Model of aging-related and cortisol induced hippocampal dysfunction". *BMC Neurosci* **10** (1): 26. doi:10.1186/1471-2202-10-26. PMID 19320982.

32. Newsholme, E.A., Leech, A.R. "Biochemistry for the Medical Sciences. John Wiley & Sons, New York, on p736.

33. Davies E. Keyon, C.J.; Fraser, R. (1985) "The role of calcium ions in the mechanism of ACTH stimulation of cortisol synthesis." Steroids 45: 557.

34. Plotsky PM, Otto S, Sapolsky RM (September 1986). "Inhibition of immunoreactive corticotropin-releasing factor secretion into the hypophysial-portal circulation by delayed glucocorticoid feedback". *Endocrinology* **119** (3): 1126–30. PMID 3015567.

35. Besedovsky, H.O.; Del Rey, A.; Sorkin, E. (1984) "Integration of Activated Immune Cell Products in Immune Endocrine Feedback Circuits." p. 200 in Leukocytes and Host Defense Vol. 5[Oppenheim, J.J.; Jacobs, D.M., eds]. Alan R. Liss, New York,.

36. Dvorak, M.; "Plasma 17-Hydroxycorticosteroid Levels in Healthy and Diarrheic Calves." British Veterinarian Journal 127: 372, 1971.

37. Besedovsky, H.O.; Del Rey, A.; Sorkin, E. (1984) "Integration of Activated Immune Cell Products in Immune Endocrine Feedback Circuits." p. 200 in Leukocytes and Host Defense Vol. 5[Oppenheim, J.J.; Jacobs, D.M., eds]. Alan R. Liss, New York,.

38. Stith RD, McCallum RE (1986). "General effect of endotoxin on glucocorticoid receptors in mammalian tissues". *Circ. Shock* **18** (4): 301–9. PMID 3084123.

39. Mikosha, A.S.; Pushkarov, I.S.; Chelnakova, I.S.; Remennikov, G.Y.A. (1991) "Potassium Aided Regulation of Hormone Biosynthesis in Adrenals of Guinea Pigs Under Action of Dihydropyridines: Possible Mechanisms of Changes in Steroidogenesis Induced by 1,4, Dihydropyridines in Dispersed Adrenocorticytes." Fiziol.[Kiev] 37: 60,.

40. Mendelsohn FA, Mackie C (July 1975). "Relation of intracellular K+ and steroidogenesis in isolated adrenal zona glomerulosa and fasciculata cells". *Clin Sci Mol Med* **49** (1): 13–26. PMID 168026.

41. Ueda Y, Honda M, Tsuchiya M, et al. (April 1982). "Response of plasma ACTH and adrenocortical hormones to potassium loading in essential hypertension". *Jpn. Circ. J.* **46** (4): 317–22. PMID 6283190.

42. Bauman K Muller J 1972 "Effect of potassium on the final status of aldosterone biosynthesis in the rat. I 18-hydroxylation and 18hydroxy dehydrogenation. II beta-hydroxylation." Acta Endocrin. Copenh. 69; I 701-717, II 718-730.

43. LaCelle PL et al. (1964) "An investigation of total body potassium in patients with rheumatoid arthritis." Proceedings of the Annual Meeting of the American Rheumatism Association, Arthritis and Rheumatism 7; 321.

44. Golf, Sw; Happel, O; Graef, V; Seim, Ke (Nov 1984). "Plasma aldosterone, cortisol and electrolyte concentrations in physical exercise after magnesium supplementation" (Free full text). *Journal of clinical chemistry and clinical biochemistry. Zeitschrift fur klinische Chemie und klinische Biochemie* **22** (11): 717–21. ISSN 0340-076X. PMID 6527092. http://toxnet.nlm.nih.gov/cgi-bin/sis/search/r?dbs+hsdb:@term+@rn+50-23-7. edit

45. Golf, Sw; Bender, S; Grüttner, J (Sep 1998). "On the significance of magnesium in extreme physical stress". *Cardiovascular drugs and therapy / sponsored by the International Society of Cardiovascular Pharmacotherapy* **12 Suppl 2**: 197–202. doi:10.1023/A:1007708918683. ISSN 0920-3206. PMID 9794094. edit

46. Wilborn, Cd; Kerksick, Cm; Campbell, Bi; Taylor, Lw; Marcello, Bm; Rasmussen, Cj; Greenwood, Mc; Almada, A; Kreider, Rb (Dec 2004). "Effects of Zinc Magnesium Aspartate (ZMA) Supplementation on Training Adaptations and Markers of Anabolism and Catabolism" (Free full text). *Journal of the International Society of Sports Nutrition* **1** (2): 12–20. doi:10.1186/1550-2783-1-2-12. PMID 18500945. PMC: 2129161. http://www.jissn.com/content/1/2/12. edit

47. Bhathena, Sj; Berlin, E; Judd, Jt; Kim, Yc; Law, Js; Bhagavan, Hn; Ballard-Barbash, R; Nair, Pp (01 Oct 1991). "Effects of omega 3 fatty acids and vitamin E on hormones involved in carbohydrate and lipid metabolism in men" (Free full text). *The American journal of clinical nutrition* **54** (4): 684–8. ISSN 0002-9165. PMID 1832814. http://www.ajcn.org/cgi/pmidlookup?view=long&pmid=1832814. edit

48. Delarue, J; Matzinger, O; Binnert, C; Schneiter, P; Chioléro, R; Tappy, L (Jun 2003). "Fish oil prevents the adrenal activation elicited by mental stress in healthy men" (Free full text). *Diabetes & metabolism* **29** (3): 289–95. doi:10.1016/S1262-3636(07)70039-3. ISSN 1262-3636. PMID 12909818. http://www.masson.fr/masson/MDOI-DM-06-2003-29-3-1262-3636-101019-ART12. edit

49. Uedo, N; Ishikawa, H; Morimoto, K; Ishihara, R; Narahara, H; Akedo, I; Ioka, T; Kaji, I; Fukuda, S (Mar 2004). "Reduction in salivary cortisol level by music therapy during colonoscopic examination" (Free full text). *Hepato-gastroenterology* **51** (56): 451–3. ISSN 0172-6390. PMID 15086180. http://www.nlm.nih.gov/medlineplus/colonoscopy.html. edit

50. Field, T; Hernandez-Reif, M; Diego, M; Schanberg, S; Kuhn, C (Oct 2005). "Cortisol decreases and serotonin and dopamine increase following massage therapy". *The International journal of neuroscience* **115** (10): 1397–413. doi:10.1080/00207450590956459. PMID 16162447. edit

51. http://www.fasebj.org/cgi/content/meeting_abstract/22/1_MeetingAbstracts/946.11

52. http://www3.interscience.wiley.com/journal/122213505/abstract

53. Hellhammer, J; Fries, E; Buss, C; Engert, V; Tuch, A; Rutenberg, D; Hellhammer, D (Jun 2004). "Effects of soy lecithin phosphatidic acid and phosphatidylserine complex (PAS) on the endocrine and psychological responses to mental stress". Stress (Amsterdam, Netherlands) **7** (2): 119–26. doi:10.1080/10253890410001728379. PMID 15512856. edit

54. Starks MA, Starks SL, Kingsley M, Purpura M, Jäger R (2008). "The effects of phosphatidylserine on endocrine response to moderate intensity exercise". *J Int Soc Sports Nutr* **5**: 11. doi:10.1186/1550-2783-5-11. PMID 18662395.

55. Vitamin C: Stress Buster Psychology today

56. Lovallo WR, Farag NH, Vincent AS, Thomas TL, Wilson MF (March 2006). "Cortisol responses to mental stress, exercise, and meals following caffeine intake in men and women". *Pharmacol. Biochem. Behav.* **83** (3): 441–7. doi:10.1016/j.pbb.2006.03.005. PMID 16631247.

57. http://cat.inist.fr/?aModele=afficheN&cpsidt=2068517

58. Robson PJ, Blannin AK, Walsh NP, Castell LM, Gleeson M (February 1999). "Effects of exercise intensity, duration and recovery on in vitro neutrophil function in male athletes". *Int J Sports Med* **20** (2): 128–35. PMID 10190775.

59. Gleeson, M (Mar 2006). "Can nutrition limit exercise-induced immunodepression?". *Nutrition reviews* **64** (3): 119–31. doi:10.1111/j.1753-4887.2006.tb00195.x. ISSN 0029-6643. PMID 16572599. edit

60. Kraemer WJ, Spiering BA, Volek JS, et al. (January 2009). "Recovery from a national collegiate athletic association division I football game: muscle damage and hormonal status". *J Strength Cond Res* **23** (1): 2–10. doi:10.1519/JSC.0b013e31819306f2. PMID 19077734.

61. Shalev, I; Lerer, E; Israel, S; Uzefovsky, F; Gritsenko, I; Mankuta, D; Ebstein, Rp; Kaitz, M (Apr 2009). "BDNF Val66Met polymorphism is associated with HPA axis reactivity to psychological stress characterized by genotype and gender interactions". *Psychoneuroendocrinology* **34** (3): 382–8. doi:10.1016/j.psyneuen.2008.09.017. PMID 18990498. edit

62. Cagnacci, A; Soldani, R; Yen, Ss (Mar 1997). "Melatonin enhances cortisol levels in aged women: reversible by estrogens" (Free full text). *Journal of pineal research* **22** (2): 81–5. doi:10.1111/j.1600-079X.1997.tb00307.x. ISSN 0742-3098. PMID 9181519. http://toxnet.nlm.nih.gov/cgi-bin/sis/search/r?dbs+hsdb:@term+@rn+50-23-7. edit

63. Wingenfeld, K; Schulz, M; Damkroeger, A; Rose, M; Driessen, M (Mar 2009). "Elevated diurnal salivary cortisol in nurses is associated with burnout but not with vital exhaustion". *Psychoneuroendocrinology*. doi:10.1016/j.psyneuen.2009.02.015. PMID 19321266. edit

64. http://diabetes.diabetesjournals.org/cgi/content/abstract/58/1/46

65. http://www.ajcn.org/cgi/content/abstract/ajcn.2008.26958v1

66. http://news.bbc.co.uk/2/hi/health/5405686.stm

67. http://www.springerlink.com/content/m226111566k24u65/

68. New Clues about Genetic Influence of Stress on Men's Health

69. Oral Contraceptive Use Impairs Muscle Gains in Young Women

70. http://www.utrc2.org/research/assets/74/commuterstress2-report1.pdf

71. Iwata, Edward (January 5, 2007). "Diet pill sellers fined $25M". *USA Today*. http://www.usatoday.com/news/washington/2007-01-04-weight-loss-pills_x.htm. Retrieved 2008-10-26.

72. Mechanism of ACTH action on adrenal cortical cells Andrew N. Margioris, M.D., and Christos Tsatsanis, Ph.D. Updated: December 4, 2006

GNU FREE DOCUMENTATION LICENSE

0. PREAMBLE

The purpose of this License is to make a manual, textbook, or other functional and useful document "free" in the sense of freedom: to assure everyone the effective freedom to copy and redistribute it, with or without modifying it, either commercially or noncommercially. Secondarily, this License preserves for the author and publisher a way to get credit for their work, while not being considered responsible for modifications made by others.

This License is a kind of "copyleft", which means that derivative works of the document must themselves be free in the same sense. It complements the GNU General Public License, which is a copyleft license designed for free software.

We have designed this License in order to use it for manuals for free software, because free software needs free documentation: a free program should come with manuals providing the same freedoms that the software does. But this License is not limited to software manuals; it can be used for any textual work, regardless of subject matter or whether it is published as a printed book. We recommend this License principally for works whose purpose is instruction or reference.

1. APPLICABILITY AND DEFINITIONS

This License applies to any manual or other work, in any medium, that contains a notice placed by the copyright holder saying it can be distributed under the terms of this License. Such a notice grants a world-wide, royalty-free license, unlimited in duration, to use that work under the conditions stated herein. The "Document", herein, refers to any such manual or work. Any member of the public is a licensee, and is addressed as "you". You accept the license if you copy, modify or distribute the work in a way requiring permission under copyright law.

A "Modified Version" of the Document means any work containing the Document or a portion of it, either copied verbatim, or with modifications and/or translated into another language.

A "Secondary Section" is a named appendix or a front-matter section of the Document that deals exclusively with the relationship of the publishers or authors of the Document to the Document's overall subject (or to related matters) and contains nothing that could fall directly within that overall subject. (Thus, if the Document is in part a textbook of mathematics, a Secondary Section may not explain any mathematics.) The relationship could be a matter of historical connection with the subject or with related matters, or of legal, commercial, philosophical, ethical or political position regarding them.

The "Invariant Sections" are certain Secondary Sections whose titles are designated, as being those of Invariant Sections, in the notice that says that the Document is released under this License. If a section does not fit the above definition of Secondary then it is not allowed to be designated as Invariant. The Document may contain zero Invariant Sections. If the Document does not identify any Invariant Sections then there are none.

The "Cover Texts" are certain short passages of text that are listed, as Front-Cover Texts or Back-Cover Texts, in the notice that says that the Document is released under this License. A Front-Cover Text may be at most 5 words, and a Back-Cover Text may be at most 25 words.

A "Transparent" copy of the Document means a machine-readable copy, represented in a format whose specification is available to the general public, that is suitable for revising the document straightforwardly with generic text editors or (for images composed of pixels) generic paint programs or (for drawings) some widely available drawing editor, and that is suitable for input to text formatters or for automatic translation to a variety of formats suitable for input to text formatters. A copy made in an otherwise Transparent file format whose markup, or absence of markup, has been arranged to thwart or discourage subsequent modification by readers is not Transparent. An image format is not Transparent if used for any substantial amount of text. A copy that is not "Transparent" is called "Opaque".

Examples of suitable formats for Transparent copies include plain ASCII without markup, Texinfo input format, LaTeX input format, SGML or XML using a publicly available DTD, and standard-conforming simple HTML, PostScript or PDF designed for human modification. Examples of transparent image formats include PNG, XCF and JPG. Opaque formats include proprietary formats that can be read and edited only by proprietary word processors, SGML or XML for which the DTD and/or processing tools are not generally available, and the machine-generated HTML, PostScript or PDF produced by some word processors for output purposes only.

The "Title Page" means, for a printed book, the title page itself, plus such following pages as are needed to hold, legibly, the material this License requires to appear in the title page. For works in formats which do not have any title page as such, "Title Page" means the text near the most prominent appearance of the work's title, preceding the beginning of the body of the text.

A section "Entitled XYZ" means a named subunit of the Document whose title either is precisely XYZ or contains XYZ in parentheses following text that translates XYZ in another language. (Here XYZ stands for a specific section name mentioned below, such as "Acknowledgements", "Dedications", "Endorsements", or "History".) To "Preserve the Title" of such a section when you modify the Document means that it remains a section"Entitled XYZ" according to this definition.

The Document may include Warranty Disclaimers next to the notice which states that this License applies to the Document. These Warranty Disclaimers are considered to be included by reference in this License, but only as regards disclaiming warranties: any other implication that these Warranty Disclaimers may have is void and has no effect on the meaning of this License.

2. VERBATIM COPYING

You may copy and distribute the Document in any medium, either commercially or noncommercially, provided that this License, the copyright notices, and the license notice saying this License applies to the Document are reproduced in all copies, and that you add no other conditions whatsoever to those of this License. You may not use technical measures to obstruct or control the reading or further copying of the copies you make or distribute. However, you may accept compensation in exchange for copies. If you distribute a large enough number of copies you must also follow the conditions in section 3.

You may also lend copies, under the same conditions stated above, and you may publicly display copies.

3. COPYING IN QUANTITY

If you publish printed copies (or copies in media that commonly have printed covers) of the Document, numbering more than 100, and the Document's license notice requires Cover Texts, you must enclose the copies in covers that carry, clearly and legibly, all these Cover Texts: Front-Cover Texts on the front cover, and Back-Cover Texts on the back cover. Both covers must also clearly and legibly identify you as the publisher of these copies. The front cover must present the full title with all words of the title equally prominent and visible. You may add other material on the covers in addition. Copying with changes limited to the covers, as long as they preserve the title of the Document and satisfy these conditions, can be treated as verbatim copying in other respects.

If the required texts for either cover are too voluminous to fit legibly, you should put the first ones listed (as many as fit reasonably) on the actual cover, and continue the rest onto adjacent pages.

If you publish or distribute Opaque copies of the Document numbering more than 100, you must either include a machine-readable Transparent copy along with each Opaque copy, or state in or with each Opaque copy a computer-network location from which the general network-using public has access to download using public-standard network protocols a complete Transparent copy of the Document, free of added material. If you use the latter option, you must take reasonably prudent steps, when you begin distribution of Opaque copies in quantity, to ensure that this Transparent copy will remain thus accessible at the stated location until at least one year after the last time you distribute an Opaque copy (directly or through your agents or retailers) of that edition to the public.

It is requested, but not required, that you contact the authors of the Document well before redistributing any large number of copies, to give them a chance to provide you with an updated version of the Document.

4. MODIFICATIONS

You may copy and distribute a Modified Version of the Document under the conditions of sections 2 and 3 above, provided that you release the Modified Version under precisely this License, with the Modified Version filling the role of the Document, thus licensing distribution and modification of the Modified Version to whoever possesses a copy of it. In addition, you must do these things in the Modified Version:

- **A.** Use in the Title Page (and on the covers, if any) a title distinct from that of the Document, and from those of previous versions (which should, if there were any, be listed in the History section of the Document). You may use the same title as a previous version if the original publisher of that version gives permission.
- **B.** List on the Title Page, as authors, one or more persons or entities responsible for authorship of the modifications in the Modified Version, together with at least five of the principal authors of the Document (all of its principal authors, if it has fewer than five), unless they release you from this requirement.

C. State on the Title page the name of the publisher of the Modified Version, as the publisher.
D. Preserve all the copyright notices of the Document.
E. Add an appropriate copyright notice for your modifications adjacent to the other copyright notices.
F. Include, immediately after the copyright notices, a license notice giving the public permission to use the Modified Version under the terms of this License, in the form shown in the Addendum below.
G. Preserve in that license notice the full lists of Invariant Sections and required Cover Texts given in the Document's license notice.
H. Include an unaltered copy of this License.
I. Preserve the section Entitled "History", Preserve its Title, and add to it an item stating at least the title, year, new authors, and publisher of the Modified Version as given on the Title Page. If there is no section Entitled "History" in the Document, create one stating the title, year, authors, and publisher of the Document as given on its Title Page, then add an item describing the Modified Version as stated in the previous sentence.
J. Preserve the network location, if any, given in the Document for public access to a Transparent copy of the Document, and likewise the network locations given in the Document for previous versions it was based on. These may be placed in the "History" section. You may omit a network location for a work that was published at least four years before the Document itself, or if the original publisher of the version it refers to gives permission.
K. For any section entitled "Acknowledgements" or "Dedications", Preserve the Title of the section, and preserve in the section all the substance and tone of each of the contributor acknowledgements and/or dedications given therein.
L. Preserve all the Invariant Sections of the Document, unaltered in their text and in their titles. Section numbers or the equivalent are not considered part of the section titles.
M. Delete any section entitled "Endorsements". Such a section may not be included in the Modified Version.
N. Do not retitle any existing section to be entitled "Endorsements" or to conflict in title with any Invariant Section.
O. Preserve any Warranty Disclaimers.

If the Modified Version includes new front-matter sections or appendices that qualify as Secondary Sections and contain no material copied from the Document, you may at your option designate some or all of these sections as Invariant. To do this, add their titles to the list of Invariant Sections in the Modified Version's license notice. These titles must be distinct from any other section titles.

You may add a section entitled "Endorsements", provided it contains nothing but endorsements of your Modified Version by various parties—for example, statements of peer review or that the text has been approved by an organization as the authoritative definition of a standard.

You may add a passage of up to five words as a Front-Cover Text, and a passage of up to 25 words as a Back-Cover Text, to the end of the list of Cover Texts in the Modified Version. Only one passage of Front-Cover Text and one of Back-Cover Text may be added by (or through arrangements made by) any one entity. If the Document already includes a Cover Text for the same cover, previously added by you or by arrangement made by the same entity you are acting on behalf of, you may not add another; but you may replace the old one, on explicit permission from the previous publisher that added the old one.

The author(s) and publisher(s) of the Document do not by this License give permission to use their names for publicity for or to assert or imply endorsement of any Modified Version.

5. COMBINING DOCUMENTS

You may combine the Document with other documents released under this License, under the terms defined in section 4 above for modified versions, provided that you include in the combination all of the Invariant Sections of all of the original documents, unmodified, and list them all as Invariant Sections of your combined work in its license notice, and that you preserve all their Warranty Disclaimers.

The combined work need only contain one copy of this License, and multiple identical Invariant Sections may be replaced with a single copy. If there are multiple Invariant Sections with the same name but different contents, make the title of each such section unique by adding at the end of it, in parentheses, the name of the original author or publisher of that section if known, or else a unique number. Make the same adjustment to the section titles in the list of Invariant Sections in the license notice of the combined work.

In the combination, you must combine any sections entitled "History" in the various original documents, forming one section entitled "History";

likewise combine any sections entitled "Acknowledgements", and any sections entitled "Dedications". You must delete all sections entitled "Endorsements."

6. COLLECTIONS OF DOCUMENTS

You may make a collection consisting of the Document and other documents released under this License, and replace the individual copies of this License in the various documents with a single copy that is included in the collection, provided that you follow the rules of this License for verbatim copying of each of the documents in all other respects.

You may extract a single document from such a collection, and distribute it individually under this License, provided you insert a copy of this License into the extracted document, and follow this License in all other respects regarding verbatim copying of that document.

7. AGGREGATION WITH INDEPENDENT WORKS

A compilation of the Document or its derivatives with other separate and independent documents or works, in or on a volume of a storage or distribution medium, is called an "aggregate" if the copyright resulting from the compilation is not used to limit the legal rights of the compilation's users beyond what the individual works permit. When the Document is included in an aggregate, this License does not apply to the other works in the aggregate which are not themselves derivative works of the Document.

If the Cover Text requirement of section 3 is applicable to these copies of the Document, then if the Document is less than one half of the entire aggregate, the Document's Cover Texts may be placed on covers that bracket the Document within the aggregate, or the electronic equivalent of covers if the Document is in electronic form. Otherwise they must appear on printed covers that bracket the whole aggregate.

8. TRANSLATION

Translation is considered a kind of modification, so you may distribute translations of the Document under the terms of section 4. Replacing Invariant Sections with translations requires special permission from their copyright holders, but you may include translations of some or all Invariant Sections in addition to the original versions of these Invariant Sections. You may include a translation of this License, and all the license notices in the Document, and any Warranty Disclaimers, provided that you also include the original English version of this License and the original versions of those notices and disclaimers. In case of a disagreement between the translation and the original version of this License or a notice or disclaimer, the original version will prevail.

If a section in the Document is entitled "Acknowledgements", "Dedications", or "History", the requirement (section 4) to Preserve its Title (section 1) will typically require changing the actual title.

9. TERMINATION

You may not copy, modify, sublicense, or distribute the Document except as expressly provided for under this License. Any other attempt to copy, modify, sublicense or distribute the Document is void, and will automatically terminate your rights under this License. However, parties who have received copies, or rights, from you under this License will not have their licenses terminated so long as such parties remain in full compliance.

10. FUTURE REVISIONS OF THIS LICENSE

The Free Software Foundation may publish new, revised versions of the GNU Free Documentation License from time to time. Such new versions will be similar in spirit to the present version, but may differ in detail to address new problems or concerns. See http://www.gnu.org/copyleft/.

Each version of the License is given a distinguishing version number. If the Document specifies that a particular numbered version of this License "or any later version" applies to it, you have the option of following the terms and conditions either of that specified version or of any later version that has been published (not as a draft) by the Free Software Foundation. If the Document does not specify a version number of this License, you may choose any version ever published (not as a draft) by the Free Software Foundation.

INDEX

Addison, Thomas, 15
Addisonian Crisis, 22, 23, 58, 81
Adrenal Crisis, 22, 47, 54, 58
Adrenal Destruction, 33, 34
Adrenal Dysgenesis, 33
Adrenal Fatigue, 83
Adrenal Gland, 15, 33, 50, 71
Adrenal Insufficiency, 15, 19, 22, 30, 33, 47–51, 54, 57, 58, 60, 65–69, 72, 73, 79, 80, 83
Adrenocorticotropic Hormone, 21, 30, 57, 98, 100, 109
Adrenoleukodystrophy, 30, 34, 71, 75–77, 79
Adrenomyeloneuropathy, 30, 72, 73, 79, 80
Aldosterone, 27, 28, 37, 47, 54, 55, 57, 62, 68–70
Amino Acids, 92, 93, 96
Autoimmune Adrenalitis, 34, 87
Autosomal, 75
Canine Hypoadrenocorticism, 45
Causes, 33, 51
Cholesterol, 33, 77, 80
Conventional-Dose Short Test, 59
Copper, 95
Corticotropin-Releasing Hormone, 98, 109
Cortisol, 28–31, 33, 37, 42, 47–49, 54, 56, 57, 60–62, 64, 65, 66, 68–70, 83, 89, 90, 92–103, 105–107, 109–111
Cortisol Stimulation, 64
Cortisone, 93, 106, 110
Diagnosis, 25, 27, 31, 37, 54, 58, 59, 65, 66, 69, 72, 74, 80
Endocrine Disorder, 15
Epidemiology, 39
Fludrocortisone, 15, 37, 45
Genetics, 33, 45, 51, 74
Glucosteroid Response Modifying Factor, 100
GNU Free Documentation License, 134
Goiter, 21
Hematopoietic Stem Cell Transplantation, 76
Hydrocortisone, 15, 21, 37, 48, 54–56, 89, 106, 107
Hypercalcemia, 23
Hyperpigmentation, 19, 21
Hypoadrenocorticism, 45
Hypocortisolism, 15, 20
Hypoglycemia, 23, 27
Hypothalamus, 20, 47, 50, 67

Impaired Steroidogenesis, 33
Insulin, 66, 92, 111
Low-Dose Short Test, 59
Melanocyte-Stimulating Hormone, 21
Myelin, 71, 72, 75
Neonatal, 73, 74
Orthostatic Hypotension, 20, 52
Pathophysiology, 74
Pituitary Gland, 20, 47, 50, 57, 66
Potassium, 27, 47, 54, 55, 69, 92–95, 97, 101
Prednisolone, 37, 45, 106, 107
Primary Adrenal Failure, 30
Prognosis, 41, 77
Prolonged-Stimulation Test, 59, 60
Sodium, 19, 27, 47, 54, 55, 62, 69, 94, 97
Stem Cell, 76, 78
Steroid Hormones, 15, 33, 47
Symptoms, 17, 19, 22, 23, 31, 33, 41, 49–52, 72, 73, 76–81, 83, 89
Testing, 29
Tetracosactide, 29, 30, 57
Treatment, 15, 37, 54, 58, 76, 77
Vitiligo, 21, 52
X-Linked, 71, 72, 74–76, 79

www.ingramcontent.com/pod-product-compliance
Ingram Content Group UK Ltd.
Pitfield, Milton Keynes, MK11 3LW, UK
UKHW021303180426
11947UKWH00015B/988